FUNDA
LAPAR
SUR

FUNDAMENTALS OF LAPAROSCOPIC SURGERY

Edited by

LAWRENCE W. WAY, M.D.
Professor and Vice Chairman
Department of Surgery
University of California, San Francisco
School of Medicine
San Francisco, California

SUNIL BHOYRUL, F.R.C.S.(Eng)
Fellow in Laparoscopic Surgery
Department of Surgery
University of California, San Francisco
School of Medicine
San Francisco, California

TOSHIYUKI MORI, M.D., Ph.D.
Associate Professor of Surgery
Chief in Minimally Invasive Surgery
First Department of Surgery
School of Medicine
Kyorin University
Tokyo, Japan

Illustrated by Terry T. Toyama, M.A.

CHURCHILL LIVINGSTONE
New York, Edinburgh, London, Melbourne, Tokyo

Library of Congress Cataloging-in-Publication Data

Fundamentals of laparoscopic surgery / edited by Lawrence W. Way,
  Sunil Bhoyrul, Toshiyuki Mori ; illustrated by Terry T. Toyama.
     p.   cm.
  Includes bibliographical references and index.
  ISBN 0-443-08991-4
  1. Endoscopic surgery.   I. Way, Lawrence, W. II. Bhoyrul, Sunil.
III. Mori, Toshiyuki.
    [DNLM: 1. Surgery, Laparoscopic. WO 500 F9808 1995]
  RD33.53.F86 1995
  617'.05 — dc20
  DNLM/DLC   95-10714
  for Library of Congress   CIP

© Churchill Livingstone Inc. 1995

Distributed in the United Kingdom by Churchill Livingstone, Robert Stevenson House, 1–3
Baxter's Place, Leith Walk, Edinburgh EH1 3AF, and by associated companies, branches,
and representatives throughout the world.

Accurate indications, adverse reactions, and dosage schedules for drugs are provided in this
book, but it is possible that they may change. The reader is urged to review the package
information data of the manufacturers of the medications mentioned.

The Publishers have made every effort to trace the copyright holders for borrowed material.
If they have inadvertently overlooked any, they will be pleased to make the necessary
arrangements at the first opportunity.

Acquisitions Editor: *Miranda Bromage*
Production Editor: *Donna C. Balopole*
Production Supervisor: *Sharon Tuder*
Desktop Coordinator: *Jo-Ann Demas*
Cover Design: *Jeannette Jacobs*

Printed in the United States of America

First published in 1995   7 6 5 4 3 2 1

▶ Contributors

Sunil Bhoyrul, B. Med. Biol., M.B. ChB., F.R.C.S.(Eng)
Fellow in Laparoscopic Surgery, Department of Surgery, University of California, San Francisco, School of Medicine, San Francisco, California

Sam H. Caravajal, M.D.
Research Fellow, Department of Surgery, University of California, San Francisco, School of Medicine, San Francisco, California

Quan-Yang Duh, M.D.
Associate Professor, Department of Surgery, University of California, San Francisco, School of Medicine, San Francisco, California

Scott D. Kelley, M.D.
Assistant Professor, Department of Anesthesia, University of California, San Francisco, School of Medicine, San Francisco, California

Toshiyuki Mori, M.D., Ph.D.
Associate Professor of Surgery and Chief in Minimally Invasive Surgery, First Department of Surgery, School of Medicine, Kyorin University, Tokyo, Japan

Sean J. Mulvihill, M.D.
Associate Professor and Chief, Division of General Surgery, Department of Surgery, University of California, San Francisco, School of Medicine, San Francisco, California

Carey Stirling, R.N.
Clinical Nurse Manager, General Surgery, Urology, Gynecology, and Liver Transplant, Operating Suite, Moffitt-Long Hospitals, University of California, San Francisco, School of Medicine, San Francisco, California

Zoltan Szabo, Ph.D., F.I.C.S.
Associate Course Director, Advanced Videoscopic Surgery Courses, Department of Surgery, University of California, San Francisco, School of Medicine, San Francisco,California.

Frank Tendick, Ph.D.
Postdoctoral Fellow, Department of Surgery, University of California, San Francisco, School of Medicine, San Francisco, California

Lawrence W. Way, M.D.
Professor and Vice Chairman, Department of Surgery, University of California, San Francisco, School of Medicine, San Francisco, California

▶ Foreword

Laparoscopic surgery has spread throughout the world and developed with unparalleled speed. The advantages it can bring to patients are such that few who have the opportunity can resist the temptation to practice laparoscopic surgery. As a result, as we now know only too clearly, the outcome for some patients is marred by avoidable complications. Emphasis has been placed upon the acquisition of manual skills training and appropriate supervision before a surgeon commences laparoscopic practice, but a comprehensive source of information concerning the basic principles and techniques has been conspicuous by its absence. Many of the books that have recently emerged provide a token chapter or so to the principles of laparoscopic surgery with the majority of the text devoted to descriptions of individual operations.

Fundamentals of Laparoscopic Surgery provides a comprehensive source of the information that laparoscopic surgeons require, whatever their field of speciality and in whichever country or type of practice they find themselves. It is authoritative and up-to-date and will guide surgeons through the apparent impenetrable forests of technology that must be confronted to gain mastery of the laparoscopic surgical environment.

The book is ideally suited to trainee laparoscopic surgeons, be they residents or consultants, and forms an ideal complement to a manual skills training course. The theoretical basis of much of the new technology is explained in a very comprehensive and readable way, but this is not a book to take down from the library shelf in the evenings. The sections on troubleshooting will make it a valuable part of the equipment in the operating room.

I congratulate the authors on the production of a such a readable and comprehensive guide to a subject that to so many is new and mysterious.

Michael J. McMahon, ChM., Ph.D., F.R.C.S.
Reader in Surgery and Consultant Surgeon
University of Leeds
Director, Leeds Institute for Minimally Invasive Therapy
The General Infirmary at Leeds
Leeds, England

▶ Preface

Fundamentals of Laparoscopic Surgery has been written to meet the needs of the newcomer to laparoscopic surgery who should have a thorough grounding in the basic principles of this technology. It will also be of value to the many other surgeons who have been performing laparoscopic cholecystectomies but have not yet had an extensive experience in more advanced laparoscopic procedures.

Unlike open surgery, many of the principles of laparoscopic surgery are not very intuitive. For example, it is critical to place the laparoscopic ports in an optimal relationship to each other or the operation may be unnecessarily difficult or even impossible. Without an explicit description of how this is done, it will take many cases before the average surgeon grasps the underlying concepts. The same can be said about complications. With every laparoscopic operation, the rate of complications has been higher than when the same procedure is performed by laparotomy. The reasons for these events have often been elusive, but enough experience is now available to understand how they come about in most cases. It turns out that the explanations constitute important generalizations about the conduct of laparoscopic surgery. Similarly, there are important points to be made about training in laparoscopic surgery, anesthesia for laparoscopic surgery, and the proper use of laparoscopic instrumentation. These subjects and many others are thoroughly covered in this concise book. We firmly believe that a knowledge of this material can shorten the learning curve for laparoscopic surgeons, thereby improving outcomes and decreasing complication rates.

The authors are all instructors in the courses in laparoscopic surgery that are conducted regularly in the Videoscopic Training Center of the University of California, San Francisco, School of Medicine. This book expresses the teaching philosophy of this unit.

Lawrence W. Way, M.D.
Sunil Bhoyrul, F.R.C.S.(Eng)
Toshiyuki Mori, M.D., Ph.D.

▶ Acknowledgments

We wish to thank the following people for their invaluable guidance and especially the instrument companies for understanding the educational goals of this book: Brian Baldrige (Synergetics), David D'Alfonso (Envision), George Deveraux (formerly of Ethicon), Christine Dickenson (Ultracision), Will Dubrul (Innerdyne), Rob Fahy (Valleylab), Mark Fighera, (United States Surgical Corporation), Tammy Folore (Valleylab), Wayne Griffis (American Surgical Technologies), Timothy E. Lippert (United States Surgical Corporation), Thomas J. Palermo (Innerdyne), John Post (Aloka), Jose Sabas (Senior Electronics Technician, University of California, San Francisco, School of Medicine), Al Smoot (Stryker), Darlyne Soong (Administrative Assistant to Dr. Way), Dave Steinbaugh (Storz), Mitchell Westcott (Maximum Design & Manufacturing), Dick Wise (Leonard Medical Inc.).

▶ Contents

1. History of Laparoscopic Surgery   1
   Toshiyuki Mori, Sunil Bhoyrul, and Lawrence W. Way

2. Principles of Instrumentation   13
   Sunil Bhoyrul, Toshiyuki Mori, and Lawrence W. Way

3. Operative Techniques   79
   Toshiyuki Mori, Sunil Bhoyrul, and Lawrence W. Way

4. Suturing   137
   Zoltan Szabo

5. Operating Room Set-Up   155
   Carey Stirling and Sunil Bhoyrul

6. Troubleshooting   169
   Quan-Yang Duh

7. Anesthetic Considerations   185
   Scott D. Kelley

8. Complications   199
   Sam H. Caravajal, Sean J. Mulvihill, and Lawrence W. Way

9.   Learning Laparoscopic Surgery   **225**
Lawrence W. Way, Sunil Bhoyrul, and
Toshiyuki Mori

10.   Future of Laparoscopic Surgery   **235**
Frank Tendick, Toshiyuki Mori, and
Lawrence W. Way

Index   **253**

History of Laparoscopic Surgery

T. Mori

S. Bhoyrul

L. W. Way

MINIMALLY INVASIVE SURGERY HAS RAPIDLY EVOLVED AS A MAJOR specialty since laparoscopic cholecystectomy was first performed in 1987. The widespread acceptance of this technique has been largely propelled by public awareness that minimally invasive surgery is associated with less pain, quicker return to normal activities, and better cosmetic results. Surgical laparoscopy, however, had been widely used by gynecologists before the explosive involvement of general surgery. In addition, other related endoscopic surgical modalities, such as arthroscopy and cystoscopy, have long been standard therapy. The growth of minimally invasive general surgery was launched by advances in imaging equipment and operating instruments. In this chapter, we review the development of minimally invasive surgical techniques and accompanying technological advances.

Development of the Endoscope

The use of endoscopy to investigate the less visible parts of the body can be traced as far back as medieval Arabia. Bozzini in 1795 is often credited with the first endoscope.[1] He used a candle as the light source to examine

the rectum and uterus. Adequate distal illumination, however, was a significant problem until Nitze in 1879 incorporated an overheated glowing piece of
platinum at the tip of his cystoscope.[2] Use of this device for gastroscopy
proved impractical because it required a constant stream of water for cooling.
Rosenheim used a miniature electric lamp for illumination in 1906, and
shortly afterward, an improved rigid instrument called Bruening's electroscope was used.[3]

Inception of Laparoscopy

The first experimental laparoscopy using dogs was described by Kelling in
1901.[4] He used a Nitze cystoscope through a large cannula to inspect the
peritoneal cavity after insufflating the abdomen with air through a needle. He
termed the technique "koelioskopie." The Swedish physician Jacobaeus suggested examining human body cavities endoscopically in 1910[5] and reported
115 examinations of the chest and abdominal cavities in 72 patients in 1911.[6]
He coined the term "laparo-thorakoskopie." Laparoscopic identification of
syphilis, tuberculosis, cirrhosis, and malignancies was reported in this clinical
series. Also in 1911, Bernheim, from the Johns Hopkins Hospital, described
experimental work and reported two examinations in humans.[7] He coined the
term "organo-scopy."

Early Clinical Experience

Although sporadic reports continued to appear in the literature, the techniques used were merely slight modifications of the original ones.[8–11] Many
innovators struggled to devise new instruments to improve the diagnostic
ability of the laparoscope. Biopsy capability was incorporated in the 1920s.[12]

The German hepatologist Kalk first described the dual trocar technique in
1929, which was the basis of later efforts in therapeutic laparoscopy.[13] He also
developed a 135° oblique view laparoscope. In 1951, Kalk published a personal series of 2000 laparoscopies without any deaths.[14]

A large series was published by Ruddock in 1937[15] detailing his personal
experience of 500 cases over a 4-year period. In this series, 39 biopsies were
taken.

Advances in Technology and Operative Techniques

The early pioneers introduced trocars and scopes directly into the peritoneal cavity. Injury to the underlying bowel and large vessels was a major problem until air was introduced into the peritoneal cavity with a needle and syringe before inserting the first trocar. An automatic pneumoperitoneum needle for safe puncture and insufflation was invented in 1918 by Goetze,[16] and in 1938 a spring-loaded needle was developed by Veress.[17] Although the Veress needle was originally devised to create a pneumothorax, the same design has been incorporated in the current insufflating needles for creating a pneumoperitoneum.

Insertion of the pneumoperitoneum needle and first trocar in the peritoneal cavity is a blind procedure and sometimes is complicated by injury to underlying structures. Because of concern about this problem, in 1974 Hasson devised a trocar with a blunt obturator, which was inserted under direct visualization of the peritoneal cavity.[18] He called his method "open laparoscopy," and it is commonly referred to today as the *Hasson technique.*

A previous attempt at safe insertion of the laparoscope was described by Decker in 1946.[19] He put the patient in the knee-chest position and inserted the scope into the pelvis through the cul-de-sac of the vagina, referring to the approach as "culdoscopy."

Although injuries to the bowel and retroperitoneal vessels were decreased by the Veress needle and pneumoperitoneum, acceptance of laparoscopy as a diagnostic method was slow because it was still considered a risky blind procedure.[20]

One of the most significant advances in the development of the laparoscope was the invention of the rod lens system by the British physicist Hopkins in 1966.[21] The rod lens worked as a light transmitter with air spaces between rod-shaped glass elements, which markedly improved resolution and brightness compared with serial glass lenses. The system is still in use today. Introduction in the 1960s of a light transmitted via fiber optic cables, the so-called cold light source, reduced considerably the risk of thermal injuries to the bowel caused by incandescent lighting.[22]

Raoul Palmer, in 1947, advocated placing patients in the Trendelenburg position after initial insufflation of the abdomen to bring the air into the pelvic cavity and urged that intra-abdominal pressure be monitored.[23] It was another two decades, however, before Kurt Semm developed an automatic insufflator that continuously monitored intra-abdominal pressure and gas flow.[24]

Semm, in Kiel, Germany, a gynecologist and engineer, has been one of the most innovative and productive researchers and clinicians in the field of laparoscopy. Many instruments and techniques devised by him are widely used in minimally invasive surgery today. He called his system *operative pelviscopy* to distinguish it from earlier attempts.[25]

Semm found that the pelvic structures could be seen better by a laparoscope with an angled lens, which constituted a considerable advance. In the early phase of operative pelviscopy, bleeding was a major problem. Semm developed a high-flow irrigation apparatus to keep the operative field clear, together with suction tubing designed not to clog with clots. To control bleeding, Semm invented the pretied suture loop (Roeder loop) and its applicator, which was designed to prevent gas leakage during the insertion of the sutures. The laparoscopic clip applier was also developed and first used in his practice. Semm refined the techniques of intra- and extracorporeal knot tying and developed needle holders and other instruments.[26,27] He developed an innovative heat transfer system, thermocoagulation, for sterilization procedures to avoid injuries related to monopolar electrocautery. Many other instruments, such as hook scissors, microscissors, cone-shaped trocars, atraumatic forceps, a uterus vacuum mobilizer, and the tissue morcellator were all invented and first used by him and his colleagues. In addition, Semm also developed a variety of laparoscopic surgical procedures, such as direct microsurgical repair of the Fallopian tube in the laparoscopic management of ectopic pregnancies, often with preservation of the affected tube; tubal sterilization by endocoagulation; salpingostomy; oophorectomy; salpingolysis; tumor reduction therapy; and frimbiolysis. He advocated laparoscopic lysis of omental adhesions, bowel suturing,[28] endometrial implant coagulation, tumor biopsy, and staging and repair of uterine perforations. He also performed the first laparoscopic appendectomy. Semm designed the Pelvitrainer to teach surgeons some of the techniques required for operative laparoscopy.[29]

The theory of lasers was conceived by Einstein in 1917 and refined by Townes and Maiman in the late 1950s and early 1960s. Laser was first used by ophthalmologists in the treatment of retinal detachment as early as the mid-1960s and shortly thereafter by otolaryngologists for vocal cord surgery.

Concerns about bowel injury from monopolar electrocautery lead many gyne-cologists to adopt lasers as an energy source for dissection and coagulation. The first clinical report describing the use of a laser in laparoscopic surgery was by Bruhat in 1979.[30] Subsequently, laser light has been widely used for dissection, coagulation, and vaporization. The claimed advantages of laser over electrocoagulation — such as better hemostasis, more precise dissection and coagulation, and decreased risk of bowel injuries, are not borne out in practice — and because they are much more expensive, lasers are rarely used by general surgeons at present (see Ch. 2).

Laparoscopic procedures were for long restricted to a single surgeon, sim-ply because the laparoscope had a single view finder. Despite articulated attachments that produced a split image, the assistant could not interact with the operator effectively because of the inefficiency and unwieldiness of the system. In 1986, this problem was solved by a computer chip TV camera attached to the laparoscope, which marked the dawn of video endoscopic surgery. More complicated procedures could be performed with active involvement of assistant surgeons. Video images of greater clarity and resolu-tion have led to greater surgical precision. Video technology has also been used to document diagnostic or operative procedures and to facilitate the training of other surgeons. Progress in imaging technology is the most signifi-cant factor in the recent increased interest in laparoscopic surgery.

Laparoscopy in General Surgery

General surgeons were slow to adopt laparoscopy for diagnosis. The exami-nation was considered incomplete because some areas of the abdominal cavity were inaccessible. Nevertheless, some pioneering surgeons recognized the value of laparoscopy and advocated its use with great enthusiasm.[31–34] Despite excellent published results, laparoscopy still did not become widely accepted, partly because computed tomography (CT) and ultrasound-guided biopsy became widely available at the same time.[35] Therefore, laparoscopy in general surgery was sometimes compared with these modalities to evaluate intra-abdominal lesions.[36] The experience showed that laparoscopy compared favorably with CT and ultrasonography in the assessment of operability of malignant tumors.[37,38] Many general surgeons were first exposed to the value of laparoscopy while assisting gynecologists in the assessment of women with atypical right lower quadrant pain. It was demonstrated that the appendix could be seen in more than 90 percent of patients. Several groups showed that laparoscopy could reduce the incidence of normal appendectomies.[39-46]

The miniature video camera, improved instrumentation, and the growing recognition that laparoscopy is effective for diagnosis and treatment led to the involvement of general surgeons in the late 1980s.

Laparoscopic Cholecystectomy

Cholecystectomy remains the treatment of choice of symptomatic gallstones despite the challenges of dissolution therapy and lithotripsy. Although these last two appeared to have a lower morbidity, their overall success rates were too low for clinical practice.[47] The advent of laparoscopic cholecystectomy coincided with the realization that dissolution and extracorporeal shock-wave lithotripsy fell short of expectations.

Filipi, Mall, and Roosma in 1985 published the first laparoscopic chole-cystectomy in an animal.[48] Exposure of the operating field, however, was inadequate with the instruments available. Furthermore, because this report preceded the introduction of video-guided laparoscopy, the operative team was unable to interact effectively. Therefore, the technique was considered unsafe and the investigation suspended. Berci and Cuschieri also proposed laparoscopic cholecystectomy several years before the first clinical case.[49]

Mouret, in Lyon, is usually credited with the first successful laparoscopic cholecystectomy in a human in 1987.[50] Mühe of West Germany, however, performed the procedure in 1985.[51] Mouret's technique of exposing the porta hepatis by forceful cephalad retraction of the gallbladder fundus is still used. Perrisat[52] and Dubois and colleagues,[53] in communication with Mouret, performed laparoscopic cholecystectomies shortly thereafter.

McKernan and Saye performed the first laparoscopic cholecystectomy in the United States in 1988,[54] followed by Reddick and Olsen,[55,56] Berci and colleagues,[57] and Ko and Airan[58] within a few months.

At first, laparoscopic cholecystectomy was confined to low-risk patients who met the following criteria: (1) symptoms consistent with biliary colic, (2) documented stones on ultrasonography or contrast radiography, (3) no evidence of common bile duct disease, (4) absence of acute cholecystitis, (5) stones less than 3.0 cm in diameter, and (6) no previous upper abdominal surgery. The indications, however, have been greatly expanded and as many as 95 percent of patients with symptomatic gallstone disease are considered candidates for this procedure today.

Initially, laser was used as an energy source for coagulation and dissection of the gallbladder in the United States. It was quickly recognized that electrocautery was cheaper and just as effective.[59]

Modern surgical advances are often the result of detailed laboratory work and careful prospective clinical trials. In the case of laparoscopic cholecystectomy, these steps were skipped, partly because of the publicity that led many American patients to demand the operation. Furthermore, many instrument companies realized the potential market in laparoscopic surgery, manufactured instruments, and hastily organized teaching courses. As a result, laparoscopic cholecystectomy was not always performed by adequately trained surgeons. In an early article, Meyers and fellow members of the Southern Surgeon Club reported that the rate of bile duct injury was high (2.2 percent) during a surgeon's first 13 laparoscopic cholecystectomies.[60] It is likely that many serious complications have not been reported.[61] Cuschieri and co-workers have cautioned against inadequate training for this procedure,[62] and it has been well shown that complications are related to the quality and frequency of training exercises.[63,64]

Laparoscopic Appendectomy

De Kok performed a laparoscopic assisted appendectomy in 1977.[65] This procedure required a minilaparotomy for removing the appendix. Semm performed the first laparoscopic appendectomy in 1983.[66] He put a suture with a straight needle through the mesoappendix and tied it for hemostasis. A Roeder loop was placed at the base of appendix, and the appendix was transected by electrocautery and removed. This was a prophylactic appendectomy performed as an ancillary procedure to a gynecologic operation.

The first laparoscopic appendectomy for acute appendicitis was described by Schreiber in 1987.[67] In his series of 70 patients with appendicitis, 7 underwent laparoscopic appendectomy for acute inflammation. In one of these patients, the appendiceal stump leaked postoperatively, which was attributed to excessive coagulation of the base of the appendix.

Laparoscopic appendectomy has not been as widely accepted as laparoscopic cholecystectomy, because open appendectomy is usually performed through a small incision and the postoperative stay is typically only a few days.

Thoracoscopic Surgery

Thoracoscopy on a human was first performed by Jacobaeus in 1911.[6] Thoracoscopy has since been used for diagnosis for recurrent pleural effusion, pleural thickening, difficult to localize intrapleural fluid, and lung biopsy. Therapeutic thoracoscopy was also first reported by Jacobeus in 1921.[68] Thoracoscopic treatment of pneumothorax was first described by Keller et al. in 1974, who applied talc poudrage through the operative thoracoscope.[69] Thoracoscopic-guided drainage of empyema cavities[70] and management of spontaneous esophageal perforation[71] have also been reported. Laser technology has also been introduced for coagulating apical blebs and obliterating the parietal pleura.[72]

Laparoscopic Surgery, Here to Stay

Laparoscopic surgery has revolutionized the practice of general surgery, and the future holds great promise. Since laparoscopic cholecystectomy was first introduced, many pioneering surgeons have been working on new procedures. Meetings and journals dealing with laparoscopic surgery have been a showcase of new procedures. In some hospitals as many as 50 percent of abdominal operations are now being done laparoscopically, and predictions have been made that 70 percent are feasible laparoscopically, without major technological advances. It is, however, obvious that what we can do is not necessarily what we should do. Although scientifically valid data comparing laparoscopic surgery with other therapeutic options are often lacking, some operations such as laparoscopic antireflux procedures have been accepted by surgeons and physicians as having such a definite role as to alter the referral pattern for surgery. Some surgeons are enthusiastic about laparoscopic colorectal surgery, whereas others are skeptical. All these procedures need to be critically appraised.

References

1. Schindler R (ed): Bozzini PH. In: Gastroscopy. University of Chicago Press, Chicago, 1937

2. Schindler R (ed): Nitze N. In: Gastroscopy. University of Chicago Press, Chicago, 1937

3. Jackson C, Jackson CL: Diseases of the Air and Food Passages of Foreign Body Origin. WB Saunders, Philadelphia, 1936

4. Kelling G: Über Oesophagoskopie, Gastroskopie und Koelioskopie. Münch Med Wochenschr 49:21, 1901

5. Jacobaeus HC: Über die Möglichkeit, die Zystoskopie bei Untersuchung seroser höhlungen Anzuwenden. Münch Med Wochenschr 57:2090, 1910

6. Jacobeus HC: Kurze Übersicht über meine Erfahrungen mit der Laparothorakoskopie. Münch Med Wochenschr 58:2017, 1911

7. Bernheim BM: Organoscopy: cystoscopy of the abdominal cavity. Ann Surg 53:764, 1911

8. Steiner OP: Abdominoscopy. Surg Gynecol Obstet 38:266, 1924

9. Stone WE: Intra-abdominal examination by the aid of the peritoneoscope. J Kans Med Soc 24:63, 1924

10. Nadeau OE, Kampmeier OF: Endoscopy of the abdomen; abdominoscopy: a preliminary study, including a summary of the literature and a description of the technique. Surg Gynecol Obstet 41:259, 1925

11. Short AR: The use of coelioscopy. Br Med J 2:254, 1925

12. Hulka JF: Textbook of Laparoscopy. p. 15. Grune & Stratton, Orlando, FL, 1985

13. Kalk H: Erfahrungen mit der Laparoskopie. Z Klin Med 111:303, 1929

14. Kalk H, Bruhl W, Burgmann W: Leitfaden der Laparoskopie und Gastroskopie. Thieme, Stuttgart, 1951

15. Ruddock JC: Peritoneoscopy. Surg Gynecol Obstet 65:623, 1937

16. Goetze O: Die Röntgedianostik bei gasgefüllter Bauchhöhle: Eine neue Methode. Münch Med Wochenschr 65:12575, 1918

17. Veress J: Neues Instrument zur Ausführung von Brust—oder Bauchpunkutionen und Pneumothoraxbehandlung. Dtsch Med Wochenschr 41:1480, 1938

18. Hasson HM: Open laparoscopy: a report of 150 cases. J Reprod Med 12:234, 1974

19. Decker A: Pelvic culdoscopy. In Meigs JV, Sturgis SH (eds): Progress in Gynecology. Grune & Stratton, Orlando, FL, 1946

20. Eisenburg J: Über eine Apparatur zur schonenden und kontrollierbaren Gasfüllung der Bauchhöhle für die Laparoskopie. Klin Wochenschr 44:593, 1966

21. Semm K: Atlas of Gynecologic Laparoscopy and Hysteroscopy. Rice AL (trans). WB Saunders, Philadelphia, 1977

22. Filipi CJ, Fitzgibons RJ, Salerno GM: Historical review: diagnostic laparoscopy to laparoscopic cholecystectomy and beyond. p. 3. In Zucker K (ed): Surgical Laparoscopy. Quality Medical Publishing, St. Louis, MO, 1991

23. Palmer R: Technique et instrumentation de la coelioscopie gynécologique. Gynecol Obstet (Paris) 46:420, 1947

24. Semm K: Operative Manual for Endoscopic Abdominal Surgery. Friederich ER (trans). Year Book Medical Publishers, Chicago, 1987

25. Semm K: History. In Sanfilippo JS, Levine RL (eds): Operative Gynecologic Endoscopy. Springer-Verlag, New York, 1989

26. Semm K: Tissue-puncher and loop-ligation—new aids for surgical therapeutic pelviscopy (laparoscopy): endoscopic intra-abdominal surgery. Endoscopy 10:119, 1978

27. Semm K: Advances in pelviscopic surgery (appendectomy). Curr Probl Obstet Gynecol 5:482, 1982

28. Semm K: The endoscopic intra-abdominal suture. Geburtshilfe Frauenheilkd 42:56, 1982

29. Semm K: Operative pelviscopy. Br Med Bull 42:284, 1986

30. Bruhat MA, Mage G, Manhes M: Use of the CO_2 laser by laparoscopy. p. 274. In Kaplan L (ed): Proceedings of the Third International Congress for Laser Surgery. Otpaz, Tel Aviv, 1979

31. Hall TJ, Donaldson DR, Brennan TG: The value of laparoscopy under local anesthesia in 250 medical and surgical patients. Br J Surg 67:751, 1980

32. Cohen HM: Peritoneoscopy in general surgery. Can J Surg 24:490, 1981

33. Cuschieri A: Laparoscopy in general surgery and gastroenterology. Br J Hosp Med 24:25, 1980

34. Berci G (ed): Endoscopy. p. 382. Appleton-Century-Crofts, East Norwalk, CT, 1976

35. Gandofi L, Rossi A, Leo P et al: Indications for laparoscopy before and after the introduction of ultrasonography. Gastrointest Endosc 31:1, 1985

36. Watt I, Anderson SD, Bell G et al: Laparoscopy, ultrasound, and computed tomography in cancer of the oesophagus and gastric cardia: a prospective comparison for detecting intra-abdominal metastases. Br J Surg 76:1036, 1989

37. Warshaw AL, Tepper JE, Shipley WU: Laparoscopy in the staging and planning of therapy for pancreatic cancer. Am J Surg 151:76, 1986

38. Possik RA, Franco EL, Pires DR et al: Sensitivity, specificity, and predictive value of laparoscopy for the staging of gastric cancer and for the detection of liver metastases. Cancer 58:1, 1986

39. Whitworth CM, Whitworth PW, Sanfillipo J, Polk HC: Value of diagnostic laparoscopy in young women with possible appendicitis. Surg Gynecol Obstet 167:187, 1988

40. Woodward A, Hemingway D: Which patients should undergo laparoscopy? letter. Br Med J 296:1740, 1988

41. Patterson-Brown S, Thompson JN, Eckersley JRT et al: Which patients with suspected appendicitis should undergo laparoscopy? Br Med J 296:1363, 1988

42. Leape L, Ramenofsky ML: Laparoscopy for questionable appendicitis. Ann Surg 191:410, 1980

43. Anteby SO, Schenker JG, Polishuk WZ: The value of laparoscopy in acute pelvic pain. Ann Surg 181:484, 1975

44. Spirtos NM, Eisenkop SM, Spirtos TW et al: Laparoscopy—a diagnostic aid in cases of suspected appendicitis. Its use in women of reproductive age. Am J Obstet Gynecol 156:90, 1987

45. Clarke PJ, Hands LJ, Gough MH, Kettlewell MC: The use of laparoscopy in the management of right iliac fossa pain. Ann R Coll Surg Engl 68:68, 1986

46. Deutsch A, Zelikovsky A, Reiss R: Laparoscopy in the prevention of unnecessary appendectomies: a prospective study. Br J Surg 69:336, 1982

47. Abd EL, Ghany AB, Holley MP, Cuschieri A: Percutaneous stone clearance of the gallbladder through an access cholecystostomy. Surg Endosc 3:126, 1989

48. Fitzgibbons RJ: Laparoscopic cholecystectomy for acute cholecystitis. Am J Gastroenterol 88:330, 1993

49. Berci G, Cuschieri A: Practical Laparoscopy. Bailliére Tindal, London, 1986

50. Perissat J, Vitale GC: Laparoscopic cholecystectomy: gateway to the future. Am J Surg 161:408, 1991

51. Mühe E: The first cholecystectomy through the laparoscope. Langenbecks Arch Chir 369:804, 1986

52. Perrisat J, Collet D, Belliard R: Gallstones: laparoscopic treatment—cholecystectomy and lithotripsy. Our own technique. Surg Endosc 4:15, 1990

53. Dubois F, Berthelot G, Levard H: Cholecystectomy par coelioscopy. Nouv Presse Med 18:980, 1989

54. McKernan JB, Saye WB: Laparoscopic general surgery. J Med Assoc Ga 79:157, 1990

55. Reddick EJ, Olsen D, Daniell J et al: Laparoscopic laser cholecystectomy. Laser Med Surg News Adv February:38, 1989

56. Reddick EJ, Olsen DO: Laparoscopic laser cholecystectomy. Surg Endosc 3:131, 1989

57. Berci G, Sackier JM, Paz-Partlow M: Laparoscopic cholecystectomy: mini-access surgery—Reality or utopia? Postgrad Gen Surg 2:50, 1990

58. Ko ST, Airan MC: Review of 300 consecutive laparoscopic cholecystectomies. Development, evolution and results. Surg Endosc 5:103, 1991

59. Zucker KA, Bailey RW, Gadacz TR, Imbembo AL: Laparoscopic guided cholecystectomy. Am J Surg 161:36, 1991

60. The Southern Surgeon Club. A Prospective analysis of 1518 laparoscopic cholecystectomies. N Engl J Med 324:1073, 1991

61. Reddick EJ, Olsen DO: Laparoscopic laser cholecystectomy: a comparison with minilap cholecystectomy. Surg Endosc 3:131, 1989

62. Cuschieri A, Berci G, McSherry CK: Laparoscopic cholecystectomy [E]. Am J Surg 159:273, 1990

63. Bailey RW, Imbembo AL, Zucker KA: Establishment of a laparoscopic cholecystectomy training program. Am Surg 57:231, 1991

64. Sackier JM: Training and education in laparoscopic surgery. p. 1. In Cuschieri A, Berci G (eds): Laparoscopic Biliary Surgery. Blackwell, London, 1990

65. De Kok H: A new technique for resecting the non-inflamed not-adhesive appendix through a mini-laparotomy with the aid of the laparoscope. Arch Chir Neerl 29:195, 1977

66. Semm K: Endoscopic appendicectomy. Endoscopy 15:59, 1983

67. Schreiber J: Early experience with laparoscopic appendectomy in women. Surg Endosc 1:211, 1987

68. Jacobaeus HC: The cauterization of adhesions in pneumothorax treatment of tuberculosis. Surg Gynecol Obstet 32:493, 1921

69. Keller R, Gutersohn J, Herzog H: The management of persistent pneumothorax by thoracoscopic procedures. Thoraxchirurgie 22:457, 1974

70. Hutter J, Harari D, Braimbridge M: The management of empyema thoracis by thoracoscopy and irrigation. Ann Thorac Surg 39:517, 1985

71. Hutter J, Fenn A, Braimbridge M: The management of spontaneous oesophageal perforation by thorascopy and irrigation. Br J Surg 72:208, 1985

72. Torre M, Belloni P: Nd:YAG laser pleurodesis through thoracoscopy: new curative therapy in spontaneous pneumothorax. Ann Thorac Surg 47:887, 1989

2

▸ Principles of Instrumentation

S. Bhoyrul

T. Mori

L. W. Way

THE REVOLUTION IN LAPAROSCOPIC SURGERY HAS BEEN MADE POSSIBLE only by the tremendous advances in instrumentation that have taken place since 1986. The aim of this chapter is to describe the important features of these new instruments that have made it possible for the surgeon to perform video endoscopic surgery. A knowledge of this material will help the surgeon to use videoscopic equipment effectively. It should allow a better understanding of the limitations of these instruments and serve as a guide to purchasing new instruments. We have not mentioned individual manufacturers. Nevertheless, we are extremely grateful to our friends in industry who have contributed to this and other chapters.

Imaging Equipment

The Laparoscope

Most laparoscopic surgery is performed with rigid laparoscopes using the rod lens system designed by Hopkins (Fig. 2-1A & B). This comprises an objective lens, which gathers a wide field of view, a series of rod lenses, an image reversal system, and an eyepiece. The Hopkins rod lens, made of quartz, replaced serial glass lenses, which reduced

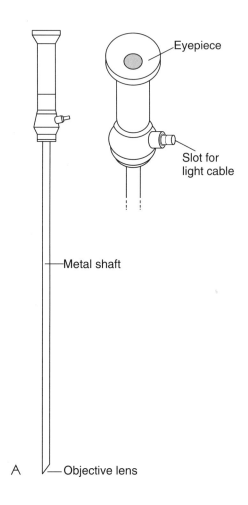

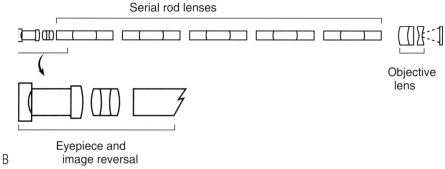

Fig. 2-1. The rigid laparoscope. **(A)** External view showing the eyepiece (to which the camera is attached), slot for insertion of light cable, metal shaft, and objective lens. **(B)** The rod lens system designed by Hopkins. *(Figure continues.)*

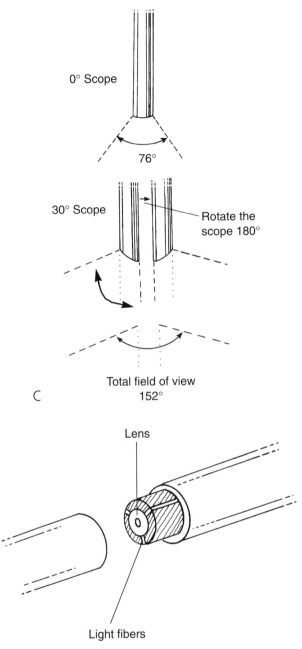

0° Scope

76°

30° Scope

Rotate the
scope 180°

Total field of view
152°

C

Lens

D   Light fibers

Fig. 2-1. *(Continued).* **(C)** Difference between a 0° (forward viewing) and 30° scope. The 0° scope has a 76° field of view. By rotating the 30° scope, one may gain a panoramic view of the abdomen. In addition, the surgeon in some situations may gain an en face view of the anatomic structure, as opposed to an oblique view with the 0° scope. **(D)** Circumferential arrangement of the light fibers around the lens train of the laparoscope provides an even distribution of light throughout the visual field.

the total amount of light transmitted as a result of reflection and absorption at each relay lens. The quartz lens absorbs relatively little light and is lined with an antireflective coating. Furthermore, being longer, it reduces the number of relay stations required.

Rigid laparoscopes come in a variety of sizes—3, 5, 7, and 10 mm—and have an option of a working channel. An intrinsic limitation of rigid scopes is the limited field of view when compared with the human eye. The human eyes, together, see a field of vision that is slightly greater than 180°. This means that we can see everything in front of us. A laparoscope, in contrast, has a much smaller field of view. Thus, the field of view of a 10-mm laparoscope is approximately 76° (some variability between manufacturers). This leads to the often cited "limited perspective" of laparoscopic surgery. The 10-mm scope without a working channel is the most commonly used laparoscope. The 5-mm scope is also commonly used for diagnostic and therapeutic procedures. They only need a 5-mm port, but because the objective lens is smaller than the 10-mm scope, the target area is also limited, even though the field of view may be as high as 90°.

A further limitation of the smaller diameter scopes is that there is proportionately less illumination of the target area. In general, 5-mm scopes have been reserved for instances when the target area is small. A key feature of laparoscopes is the angulation of the objective lens, which as Figure 2-1C shows, can be used to provide a panoramic view of the operating field. A laparoscope without angulation (i.e., a 0° lens) of the objective lens is referred to as a *forward viewing scope*. The earlier models with angulated lens had a significant loss of light, but the image on modern versions is bright. Although angled scopes are more difficult to use, they can contribute significantly to the procedure, by allowing better viewing from angles that cannot be reached by conventional forward viewing scopes, thus allowing the surgeon to look into less accessible areas (e.g., behind the esophagus) or look at a structure from a more satisfactory angle (e.g., en face view of Calot's triangle during laparoscopic cholecystectomy). An en face view of the operative site is obtained by placing the objective lens of the scope perpendicular to the target tissue. In many instances (e.g., operating over the inguinal canal), this is only possible by using an angled scope. In other situations, the port for the laparoscope can be positioned to allow an en face view using the 0° scope. A 45° and 50° angulation is also available.

The lens system of the laparoscope is surrounded by a series of fiber-optic bundles, which transmit light from the light source to the field of view (i.e., the operative site) (Fig. 2-1D). The circumferential arrangement of these fibers leads to an even distribution of light throughout the field of view. The laparoscope has a proximal slot for the insertion of the light cord. In angulated scopes, this slot is usually (but not always) exactly opposite the direction of the lens. Therefore, if the slot and cord are held upward, the lens points downward, giving the view of looking down.

The difference between the ambient temperature and the intra-abdominal temperature often leads to misting of the objective lens of the laparoscope. This problem may be overcome by warming the scope before insertion, or by wiping the lens with povidone iodine or commercially available antifogging solutions, which usually contain isopropyl alcohol. The temperature difference across the objective lens is exacerbated by connecting the insufflation gas through the same port as the laparoscope. In our experience, connecting the insufflator tubing to a different port reduces considerably the incidence of misting.

Another common problem is the blinding of the laparoscope with a spray of blood, often as a blood vessel is accidentally cut. This usually necessitates removal of the laparoscope to clean the lens, during which time the operating field is quickly covered in blood. One attempt to overcome this problem has been to incorporate a windscreen washer-type device on the surface of the lens, which is activated either by a button on the camera head or by injecting a stream of saline through the scope itself.

Fiber-optic scopes, although used routinely by gastroenterologists, have not been widely accepted as an alternative to the rigid laparoscopes in laparoscopic surgery. With these scopes, each fiber sees only a small part of the visual field, so that the final image is a summation of the images seen by all the fibers. This feature intrinsically limits the resolution of the image, which has not matched that produced by a rigid Hopkins lens system. Fiber-optic scopes also have a much smaller field of view than the human eye, and furthermore, the field of view is smaller than a laparoscope of comparable diameter. The advantages of fiber-optic scopes are their flexibility and the ability to change the viewing angle. Therefore, they are especially useful for procedures in which these features are imperative, such as choledocoscopy and occasionally thoracoscopy. An interesting application of fiber-optic technology is a 2-mm fiber-optic scope that allows inspection of the peritoneal cavity through the small bore of the insufflation needle.[1] If the resolution of fiber-optic scopes improves, this technology may be used in more situations.

The Camera Unit

One Chip or Three Chips?

Most camera systems are separate from the laparoscope. Although integrated camera/laparoscope systems are available, they do not afford the flexibility of varying the angulation or size of the laparoscope during a procedure. The most important part of a camera is the silicon chip that is responsible for receiving the image from the laparoscope. This chip is termed the *charge-coupling device (CCD)* and is divided into thousands of light-sensitive squares (elements). As a series of photons of light strike an element, an electronic signal is generated, which is sent to a processor and reassembled to form a television image. A color image may be constructed in several ways. In the classic one-chip camera, a color grid is placed in front of the CCD to divide the incoming light into its three primary colors (red, green, and blue). Each element of the CCD senses either red, green, or blue light, and the resulting electronic signal is reconstructed to form a color image. In a three-chip camera, the incoming light is first passed through a prism to divide it into its three primary colors. Three separate CCDs are then placed to detect each primary color. This system leads to an image of much higher resolution than the one-chip camera but is also more expensive and may have problems with distorted colors that are due to misalignment of the prism with the CCDs. A method of improving the resolution of the one-chip camera is to place a strobe in front of the CCD, which exposes the CCD to red, green, and blue light sequentially. This also improves resolution of one-chip cameras. Manufacturers often describe the resolution of a camera in terms of the number of horizontal lines into which the final image is divided on the television screen. The more the lines, the greater the resolution. Hence, the resolution of the original one-chip camera was approximately 470 lines, while that of the three-chip cameras is in the region of 750 lines.

An important point to remember when purchasing a system is that other important determinants of image quality are rarely quantified, such as the type of signal transmitted by the camera (see below), signal-to-noise ratio, and edge enhancement. The greatest source of noise is so-called thermal noise, which is an aberrant signal that results from electrons on the CCD that vibrate (and thus generate a signal) in response to heat. There are important design features that reduce the amount of thermal noise, such as placing most of the heat-generating components of the camera in a camera console box distant from the CCD on the hand-held camera unit. Nevertheless, other sources of heat (surgeon's hand, sterilization process, prolonged use) may cause varying amounts of noise with different systems. The most reliable way, therefore, of comparing two systems is to actually try them out against each other. Finally, it should be remembered that the resolution of the TV monitor should be as high as the resolution of the camera, although in practice, the camera and monitor are usually purchased as systems from the manufacturer.

Iris, White Balance, and Gain

The camera head is connected to a distant console box, which receives and processes the electronic signal from the microchip(s) in the camera. This box also contains the appropriate dials for controlling the power supply, iris (manual or automatic), color calibration (white balance), and gain.

The amount of light processed by the camera is adjusted by an iris. This is usually set automatically, but if reflections from instruments and peritoneum lead to an inappropriate darkening of the visual field, a manual override of the iris is possible. The original iris was a manual iris similar to that in front of the human lens. The newer systems have an electronic iris linked to the CCD itself, which controls overall illumination of the picture by a feedback mechanism. This is a more sensitive means of controlling the brightness of the field, so the sudden darkening and relighting of the field that may occur with the older systems—when a reflective surface (e.g., metal instrument) is placed in front of the laparoscope—is less likely to occur. Nevertheless, cameras from different manufacturers vary greatly in the exact way in which the luminescence is controlled. Some designs use the amount of light in the center of the visual field to control the luminescence, whereas another typical design divides the entire visual field into nine equal parts and gives a different emphasis to each of the nine parts to the amount of control it has on the overall luminescence. The end result in the different systems leads to significant differences in picture quality among manufacturers.

Before each operation, the camera's color system should be calibrated by focusing on a white surface and activating the white balance feature of the camera box. Activating this white balance switch allows the camera to adjust its parameters for red, green, and blue, on the assumption that the white surface contains equal amounts of these three primary colors. It is important, therefore, that a *pure white* surface is chosen (typically a clean swab) and that the process of white balancing takes place with the light source and laparoscope connected to the camera, because these define the operating conditions of the system. *Gain* refers to the amount of light from the visual field that is processed by the camera. A high-gain setting will therefore increase the amount of light processed by the camera (by amplifying the signal), but it may also lead to a poorer resolution (a grainy picture) and some loss of color accuracy, as the noise in the signal is also amplified.

Types of Signal

Composite Video, Y/C, or RGB

The simplest type of signal transmitted by the camera box to the monitors and recording equipment is a composite video signal. There is, however, a loss of image quality in the cables used to transmit this signal and also in the microprocessors used to interpret the signal. The next advance, therefore, has been to split the image into several components, enabling the monitor or recorder to reconstitute a final image of higher quality than a composite video image. The first such split was to divide the image into its components of brightness and color, the *Y/C* signal. Reconstitution of this signal by a suitably equipped video recorder leads to a high-quality image termed a *super-VHS* image. Another method of improving image quality is to transmit the color signal as its component red, green, and blue signals (the *RGB* signal), which are then restructured by the receiving monitor or recorder as a color picture. The newer camera boxes have an array of different signal outputs at the back, allowing a choice of signal and also the ability to split the signals (e.g., an RGB signal to the main monitor, a super-VHS signal to the video recorder, and a composite video signal to the accessory monitor, thus allowing the surgeon to view the highest quality RGB signal while recording a super-VHS signal).

Digital Processing

A further refinement in image processing has been the introduction of digital processing of the signal transmitted by the CCD in the camera head. The original analog signal is transmitted as a continuous waveform that is infinitely variable. Its intrinsic limitation is that any distortion to the waveform makes it impossible to reproduce exactly the signal transmitted. This distortion occurs in the cables and electronics used to process and transmit the signal and also occurs in the presence of interference from other signals. A digital signal is expressed as a discrete series of numbers (expressed in binary), so that reproduction is more likely to be exact. With digital audio signals, as a safeguard against the loss of individual numbers (distortion), the signal is encoded so that, for example, every fourth number is the sum of the previous three numbers. Such coding of the signal allows the processor to recalculate the original signal in the face of limited distortion. This coded signal, however, has not yet been incorporated into digital video signals. The final image, using a digital camera, has been compared to the improvement in sound quality from digital audio compact disc players compared with analog record players. This comparison, however, is not strictly accurate; with the current digital cameras, only the processing of the signal occurs in digital format, whereas the transmission of the signal from camera head to camera box and also from the camera box to the monitor occurs in the conventional analog form. Distortion of the signal during transmission is still possible, especially if the signal is transmitted through a video recorder before it reaches a monitor. The improvement in image quality produced by using a digital camera may therefore be negated by the arrangement of the monitors and recording equipment and also by distortion in the cables used for transmission of the signal.

An important practical issue is to make sure that the monitor/recording equipment is compatible with the signal transmitted from the camera box. For example, if an RGB digital output is chosen from the camera console box, then the monitor must have the appropriate RGB digital input, and the RGB digital switch must be selected. The technique for operating the camera is discussed in Chapter 3 and should be reviewed.

Second Camera

A second camera system is commonly used during procedures within the lumen of an organ system (e.g., common bile duct exploration and intragastric surgery). This usually requires a separate camera and monitor system to be wheeled into the operating room, although signal mixers are available that obviate the need for a second monitor by providing two images within the same monitor (the split screen image).

Stereoscopic imaging systems for use in laparoscopic surgery are considered in Chapter 10.

Sterilization

Sterilization of a camera head and cable unit may be performed in several ways and depends ultimately on the manufacturer's recommendations. The options are gas sterilization (e.g., ethylene oxide); soaking in a disinfectant solution such as glutaraldehyde or 100 percent alcohol; using one of the commercially available chemical sterilization systems (e.g., the Steris system, which is a portable sterilization unit that uses peroxyacetic acid, steam, and pressure to sterilize a camera unit in 30 minutes); or not sterilizing the camera, but merely covering it with a sterile plastic drape during use.

Sterilization is a potentially damaging process, especially if it introduces a troublesome film of moisture between the camera and connecting piece for the laparoscope. The preferred method of sterilization thus depends on the specifications and warranty agreement with the manufacturer. A convenient regimen is to gas sterilize a camera unit overnight and then to use the Steris system between cases. Soaking a camera in solution between cases is a form of disinfection rather than sterilization and therefore may not be considered entirely satisfactory by some. The alternative method of draping the camera may be cumbersome and has the disadvantage of not permitting a sterile swap of the laparoscope (e.g., when changing from a 0° to a 30° or from a 10- to a 5-mm laparoscope) during the procedure. The recommended method of sterilization should be an important consideration for a hospital when purchasing a camera unit, especially if only one or two cameras are available in the operating suite.

The Monitor

To take advantage of the high resolution of the more advanced cameras, a high-resolution monitor is required. Conventional TV monitors project the image as 525 horizontal lines (625 in the United Kingdom or other countries that use the PAL standard). High-resolution monitors use 700 lines, suitable for the three-chip cameras. The important variables that affect the quality of the image on the computer monitor are the horizontal scan rate and the dot pitch. The horizontal scan rate refers to the rate at which an electron beam travels across the screen and therefore affects the number of times in a second that a monitor repaints the screen (the refreshing rate). Although this rate is variable with computer monitors, the scan rate of video monitors is determined by national and international broadcasting standards (PAL and National Television Standards Council [NTSC]). Some potentially major improvements in the quality of the image on a video monitor are therefore limited by the current adherence of manufacturers to these broadcasting standards. The dot pitch is the distance (in millimeters) between the phosphor dots on a television screen. The smaller the distance, the sharper the image. A distance of less than 0.28 mm is considered optimal. As mentioned earlier, most monitors are purchased as part of a system from a manufacturer. It is important, however, to consider the potential for improvement in image quality by choosing an appropriate monitor and to discuss this with the distributor at the time of purchase. Some monitors are designed to receive either a composite video signal or the higher quality Y/C or RGB signals. The type of signal received is determined by the signal output of the camera box. As previously discussed, some camera systems can transmit more than one type of signal, so that different quality signals may be selectively sent to the monitor, the accessory monitor, and the recording equipment. One must select the appropriate signal input switch on the monitors and recording equipment.

An important practical issue is that of signal termination. Because the signal transmitted from the camera may be sent in series to various sources (typically, two monitors and a video recorder), the monitor may or may not be the last item in the transmission of the signal. If a monitor is the last item, the signal must be terminated by passing it through a resistor. In practice, this is done by switching a termination switch behind the monitor from off to on. Failure to do so may result in the display of a ghost image on the monitor. Some of the newer monitors can recognize and automatically terminate the signal, and they do not have a termination switch.

Light Source

The light source typically consists of a 300-watt fan-cooled xenon lamp, the intensity of which can be varied, connected to the laparoscope by a fiber-optic cable (the light cord). The light is transmitted along the shaft of the laparoscope by a set of fiber-optic bundles arranged circumferentially around the Hopkins lens (Fig. 2-1D). This arrangement of placing the light source distant from the laparoscope was designed to prevent overheating at the tip of the laparoscope and is referred to as a *cold light source*. Nevertheless, some heating does occur, so it is important to avoid prolonged direct contact between the tip of the laparoscope and the patient, operating staff, or drapes. Damage to the fiber-optic bundles in the light cord reduces the amount of light at the tip of the laparoscope. It is therefore important periodically to inspect the light cord by shining a low-intensity light through it and projecting the light against a wall. Black spots in the projected image represent broken fibers. It is recommended that if more than 20 percent of the fibers are broken, the cord should be replaced.[2]

Recording Equipment

The ability to record laparoscopic procedures provides the ideal opportunity for surgical audit in this new and controversial field. It enables the surgeon to review his or her own operative technique and to review a case in detail if complications arise.

There are two main types of recording: continuous and still pictures. Continuous documentation of the procedure is made possible by attaching a video recorder to the imaging system. Although not widely used, RGB analog and RGB digital video recorders are available and currently produce the highest quality images. Still pictures may be taken during the procedure by attaching a 35-mm camera directly to the eyepiece of the laparoscope. This is cumbersome and often impractical; therefore, video printers and slide makers are commercially available. These printers and slide makers receive their image directly from the camera console box. When activated, an image is transmitted from the camera to the slide maker or video printer. The image is then processed and, in the case of a slide maker, exposed to a 35-mm color slide film, which may be processed and developed in a conventional manner. A video printer will process and develop the image and produce an instant color print without a stored negative film. Digitized images may also be recorded and stored in binary format, allowing manipulation of the image with a computer. These systems are relatively expensive ($10,000 to $15,000). A limitation of still pictures taken from the camera box is that they are pictures of a television image, which has already been divided into a number of lines, rather than a direct photograph. The quality of the image is therefore much poorer than a direct photograph, and this is especially apparent when the images are projected on a large screen.

Creating and Maintaining the Operating Space (Exposure)

The normal peritoneal cavity is merely a potential space. A large space therefore, has to be created, to enable the surgeon to displace the viscera, to view the operative field, and to manipulate instruments. Gaseous, liquid, and mechanical distension of the abdomen have been used, but gaseous distension is the most popular. This may be done by making a hole in the abdominal wall and lifting it to allow room air into the peritoneal cavity or by instilling a gas, under pressure, into the peritoneum. The latter method is currently the most popular, because it is easy and allows uniform distension of the peritoneal cavity.

Choice of Gas

The ideal gas used for creating a pneumoperitoneum should be biologically inert, absorbed harmlessly and rapidly into the bloodstream (so that it does not persist in the peritoneum after the procedure) and not support combustion. Carbon dioxide, although not inert, is currently the most widely used gas, despite some complications with prolonged use (see Ch. 8). Alternatives include helium and nitrous oxide. Nitrous oxide has a lower absorption into the bloodstream and is therefore recommended only for short procedures. It also has the potential to support combustion. Medical grade carbon dioxide is inexpensive and supplied in portable tanks that fit conveniently to the side of most instrument carts. Some recent work suggests the desirability of warming the gas to prevent hypothermia in elderly patients.[3]

Insufflator

An insufflator (Fig. 2-2) is designed to deliver gas for establishing and maintaining the pneumoperitoneum. In addition to the delivery of gas, insufflators have the ability to control the maximal flow rate of the gas and the pressure of gas within the abdomen. The insufflator has an inlet valve for connection to a gas tank and an outlet port from which sterile plastic tubing is passed to the patient and is used to deliver the gas.

Flow Rate

The flow of gas is controlled either in a stepwise fashion (low, medium, or high) or preset by a dial in liters/minute. Low flow rate is 1 L/min, medium flow is 2 to 3 L/min, and high flow is greater than 4 L/min. The newer insufflators allow the exact flow rate to be set and usually offer flow rates of up to 10 L/min. A flow rate of 1 L/min is used in the initial instillation of gas when establishing a pneumoperitoneum in the blind technique (see Ch. 3). A digital flow rate indicator is present on most machines. Once the desired intra-

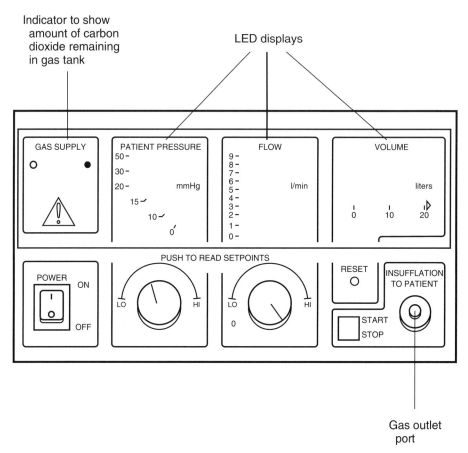

Fig. 2-2. A typical insufflator with dials that control the intra-abdominal pressure and flow rate.

abdominal pressure is achieved, a continual display of a flow rate greater than 1 L/min is indicative of a leak from the system, most commonly from one of the cannula sites. High-flow insufflators are available, which deliver flow rates of up to 20 L/min. These high-flow insufflators are often used during prolonged laparoscopic procedures with five or more trocar sites, during which there is often significant loss of gas. Although a standard insufflator can usually keep up with this loss, the high flow rate insufflator has the potential advantage of being able to restore the lost pneumoperitoneum much more rapidly. This feature is useful when the surgeon uses an irrigation device, which depletes the pneumoperitoneum. An important point to consider, however, is that the maximal flow rate depends also on the impedance to flow as it does on the delivery of gas by the insufflator. *Flow is proportional to the delivery pressure and inversely proportional to the impedance.* A simple test is to connect the insufflator tubing to the gas port of an open cannula and dangle the cannula in midair. One can now assess the maximal flow rate through this delivery system (typically about 9 L/min). In practice, this is often less than the maximal flow capability of the insufflator. This means that it is usually not possible to increase the flow with a high-flow insufflator. The maximal impedance to flow is usually in the inlet valve of the cannula. Placing a large instrument through the cannula causes a further impedance to flow. In these circumstances, it is fruitless to attempt to increase the delivery of gas by connecting to a high-flow insufflator. Higher flow may result if the delivery tubing is connected to a large cannula (e.g., 10 to 12 mm) that only has a small instrument (4- to 5-mm diameter) passing through it. Alternatively the delivery tubing may be connected to more than one cannula, using a Y-adapter.

Pressure

The pressure monitor reflects the total resistance to the instillation of gas. Therefore, in addition to the pressure within the abdomen, the reading reflects the impedance to flow within the delivery apparatus (connecting tubing and Veress needle or cannula). The pressure reading only equals intra-abdominal pressure when the flow rate approaches zero. At higher flow rates, the pressure monitor actually measures the pressure within the delivery apparatus. The surgeon should therefore remember that a high intra-abdominal pressure reading will be inaccurate if there is a high resistance to flow in the delivery apparatus, or if that reading is taken at a time of high gas flow. Once the preset pressure is achieved, the insufflator is designed to halt the delivery of gas and to recommence when the pressure falls below the preset level. In this, way the intra-abdominal pressure is maintained at a constant desired level throughout the procedure. Most insufflators have an alarm system that sounds when the pressure exceeds the level preset by the surgeon.

In addition to indicators for the intra-abdominal pressure and the flow rate, the insufflator has an indicator to show the total volume of gas delivered and a dial to show the amount of gas left within the gas tank.

Veress Needle–Blind Technique

A Veress needle (Fig. 2-3) is currently the device most commonly used for gaining access to the peritoneal cavity before insufflation. This needle has a

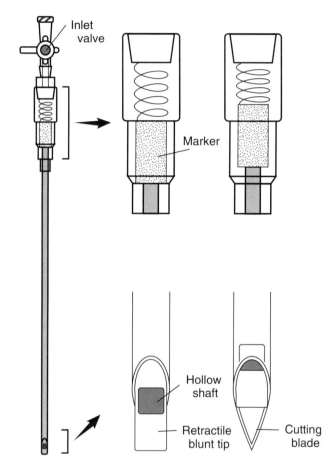

Fig. 2-3. Veress needle. Note the blunt tip that retracts on contact with tissue, to reveal a cutting blade. A marker on the handpiece also retracts, to indicate that the cutting blade is exposed.

blunt obturator, which retracts on contact with solid tissue to reveal a cutting tip. A marker on the handpiece moves upward as the obturator retracts to expose the cutting tip. Once the peritoneal cavity is entered, gas may be instilled through the hollow shaft of the needle. The needle is then removed, and a trocar/cannula is inserted through the same site. This method of peritoneal access is referred to as the *blind or closed technique* (discussed in Ch. 3).

The Trocar-Cannula Apparatus

A trocar is, strictly speaking, the cutting obturator within a cannula. In practice, the term *trocar* is commonly used by surgeons to describe the whole trocar-cannula apparatus.

Once the pneumoperitoneum is established, a cannula must be inserted to allow the passage of the laparoscope and operating instruments into the abdomen. Earlier models had multiple channels for the insertion of the laparoscope and instruments through the same cannula. With the advent of procedures more complex than diagnostic laparoscopy, it has become standard practice to use a single channel cannula for the laparoscope and separate cannulas for the working instruments. An illustration of a typical disposable trocar-cannula apparatus is shown in Figure 2-4A. This consists of a cutting obturator (the trocar) and a working cannula. The entire apparatus is inserted through the abdominal wall into the peritoneum. As a safety feature, most disposable cannulas are equipped with a plastic sleeve, which automatically covers the cutting obturator once it has pierced the abdominal wall. Alternatively, some devices automatically retract the sharp trocar into the shaft of the cannula after the trocar has pierced the abdominal wall. Reusable cannulas (Fig. 2-4B) do not have this safety feature. The presence of this "safety feature" may not prevent a trocar-related injury,[4] for two reasons. First, the plastic sleeve that covers the trocar may get caught up in the peritoneum, leaving the cutting edges of the trocar dangerously exposed within the abdominal cavity, with a subsequent risk of visceral or vascular injury. Second, the speed at which the safety shield snaps into place may be exceeded by the speed at which the trocar enters the abdominal cavity and pierces an adjacent viscus or vascular structure. This risk is higher, the greater the force of insertion, and also in the presence of adhesions, which are likely to bring structures such as bowel close to the anterior abdominal wall. No empirical evidence indicates that the safety shield reduces the incidence of complications during trocar insertion. The use of a disposable trocar-cannula apparatus, therefore, *does not guarantee safety.*

In addition to the trocar-cannula apparatus, there is the option of securing the cannula to the abdominal wall with a fascial thread that anchors the cannula to the abdominal wall by screwing into the fascial layers. As an alternative, some manufacturers use an adhesive patch that anchors the cannula to the skin

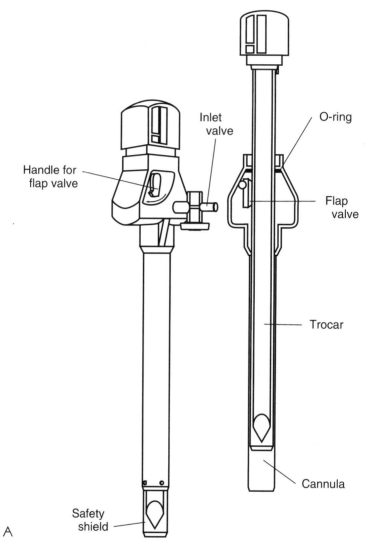

Fig. 2-4. (A) A typical disposable trocar and cannula apparatus. *(Figure continues.)*

of the abdomen. Once the trocar-cannula apparatus is successfully inserted into the abdominal cavity, the trocar is removed to leave a cannula in situ.

The cannula always contains a valve (Fig. 2-4) to prevent the loss of pneumoperitoneum when no instrument is in place. Some cannulas have a lever to hold open this valve in special circumstances, such as the removal of specimens

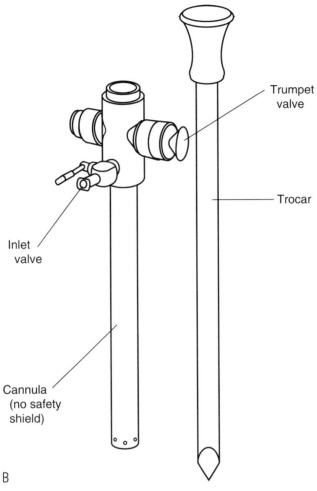

Trumpet
valve

Trocar

Inlet
valve

Cannula
(no safety
shield)

B

Fig. 2-4 *(Continued).* **(B)** Reusable trocar and cannula. Note the trumpet valve and absence of safety shield.

or suture needles, or more commonly the hook-shaped electrodes of electro-cautery devices. The cannula also contains an O-ring, which fits around an instrument and maintains the pneumoperitoneum when an instrument is in place. A second O-ring (known as a reducer) may be attached if an instrument smaller than the range of diameters covered by the original O-ring is to be inserted through the cannula. This reducer is often a simple piece of rubber with a hole of 3.5, 4.5, 5.5, or 10.5 mm in the center. The surgeon should choose a reducer valve 0.5 mm smaller than the diameter of the instrument to secure an airtight seal. Cannulas are available in a wide range of diameters (3 to 33 mm), but the most commonly used sizes are 5, 10, and 12 mm. Most commercially available cannulas follow these design principles. In a newer design, the cutting obturator has been replaced by a blunt radially expanding plastic obturator.[4a]

Reusable trocars and cannulas have a few important design differences. First, a spring-loaded trumpet valve is used to prevent air loss when no instrument is in place; second, the obturator (trocar) may dull with repeated use; and third, the apparatus is radiopaque (in contrast with the radiolucent disposable cannulas). Reusable cannulas are also available with flap valves, whch are more convenient to use than the trumpet valves.

Hasson Cannula (Open Laparoscopy)

Reports of visceral and vascular injury using the blind method of trocar insertion have led some surgeons to insert the first trocar using modifications of the Hasson cannula (Fig. 2-5) in the open laparoscopy technique. The Hasson cannula (designed by the contemporary American gynecologist, Harrith M. Hasson) and its many modifications consist of a cannula with an olive-shaped sleeve and a blunt trocar. The olive-shaped sleeve acts as a plug preventing gas leakage and is also mounted with two wings to which sutures may be tied, securing the cannula to the abdominal wall fascia. The modifications to the Hasson cannula center mainly on the method of securing the cannula to the abdominal wall. The trocar is removed to leave a wide-bore cannula through which gas may be rapidly insufflated.

Anterior Abdominal Wall Retraction Systems

As an alternative to the use of gas insufflation, devices for mechanical retraction of the anterior abdominal wall are available to create and maintain the operating space. The avoidance of the complications that are due to pneumoperitoneum was the impetus for the development of such devices.

These devices depend on either a metallic arm, circular device, T-bar, or wire holder that is either attached to the inner abdominal wall or just the skin. Usually, a second metallic arm is attached to the operating table, which provides the lifting force on the abdominal component of the device. The devices may be operated by simple traction or by a hydraulic or

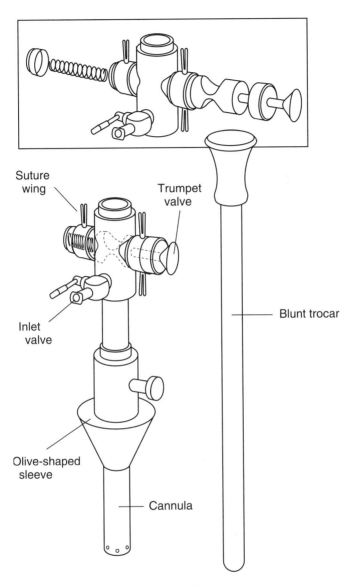

Fig. 2-5. Reusable Hasson cannula. Note the blunt trocar, olive-shaped sleeve, and wings to which sutures tied into the abdominal fascia may be attached. Variations in the Hasson cannula center mainly on the design of the sleeve and suture wings.

motorized lifting system. Such a device is shown in Figure 2-6. Insertion of the device, in some cases, may require the use of a cannula and low-pressure pneumoperitoneum.

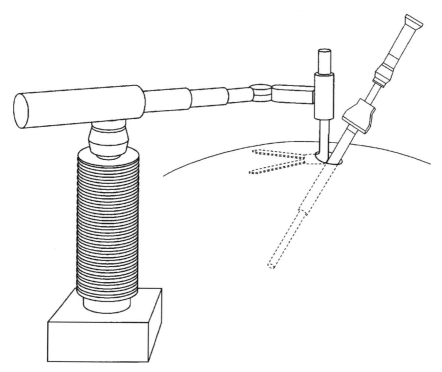

Fig. 2-6. Abdominal wall retraction device. Note the hydraulic arm attached to the operating table and lifting arm with intra-abdominal fan retractor. Laparoscope shown inserted through same site as the lifting fork.

This method of creating the operating space has the advantage of not needing an airtight seal around the sites of instrument insertion, so conventional instruments may be used.[5] This is particularly helpful in areas such as laparoscopic colorectal surgery, where conventional instruments (e.g., sponge sticks, Babcock clamps, needle holders) may offer a wider range of technical possibilities than specially designed laparoscopic instruments alone. Furthermore, more than one instrument may be inserted through a single site, avoiding the need for multiple trocar incisions. The disadvantage of the currently available devices is that they produce a tent-like space to work within, rather than the dome-shaped displacement of the abdominal wall and *viscera* produced by gas insufflation. This feature makes the devices difficult to use if the site of pathology is unknown before insertion of the device and also reduces the total working space when compared to a pneumoperitoneum. This has made the current devices unattractive for widespread use by laparoscopic surgeons. In addition, greater patient discomfort has been reported with these devices, as a result of applying so much force to the relatively small area of contact of the retractor.[6]

Performing the Surgery

Operating Instruments

Laparoscopic instruments differ from those used in open surgery, especially in their length and incorporation of many more mechanical parts. Surgeons need to understand how best to use these instruments to develop skills in videoscopic surgery.

Disposable Versus Reusable Instruments

Although most instruments used for conventional surgery are used over and over again, many of the instruments for laparoscopic surgery are made of plastics that cannot be sterilized after a single use. Manufacturers claim that the main reason for this is that current plastic molding technology allows complex instrument parts to be mass produced cheaply, hence reducing the unit cost of the instrument. Indeed, many laparoscopic instruments contain highly engineered components. A disposable grasper, for example, costs six to seven times less than a comparable reusable instrument. Furthermore, to market a product as reusable, the regulatory bodies in the United States require proof that the instrument can be repeatedly sterilized. Sterilization of laparoscopic instruments, with their many small parts, may also be difficult and time-consuming. An advantage of using some disposable instruments in laparoscopic surgery, for which instrument design is rapidly evolving (e.g., stapling and anastomosis devices), is that it allows the surgeon to use the most modern version of the instruments available, rather than to invest in a reusable instrument that may soon be obsolete. Disposable cutting instruments (e.g., scissors and trocars) also have the merit of always being sharp, in contrast with reusable versions that dull with repeated use. A major attraction of disposable instruments to surgeons is that, being new, they nearly always work. The earlier reusable instruments were often fragile and broke unpredictably. The most modern reusable instruments are probably more reliable but correspondingly more expensive.

The use of disposable instruments is partly responsible for the higher cost of laparoscopic procedures compared with open procedures. Some manufacturers have addressed this issue by making instruments with a combination of disposable and reusable components. Nevertheless, the main impetus for using reusable instruments comes from hospitals increasingly concerned with the overall higher cost of disposable instruments. The actual cost depends on the procedure but is considerably higher for operations that involve the use of disposable laparoscopic clip appliers, staplers, and linear cutting and anastomosis devices, which are often $200 to $400 per instrument. While the cost of disposables in a laparoscopic cholecystectomy may add $400 to $500 to the cost of the procedure,[7] using disposable equipment to perform a laparoscopic hysterectomy can add $1235 to $1635.[8] These costs are passed on to the patient with additional charges (a markup) imposed by the hospital.

The individual surgeon's ultimate choice of disposable or reusable instrument should take into account the performance of the instrument, its likely frequency of use, manufacturer backup and upgrade ability, and the actual cost of the instrument.

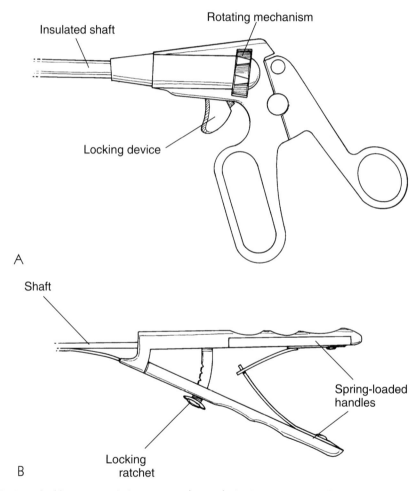

Fig. 2-7. A typical laparoscopic instrument. **(A & B)** The handle and shaft. The most common handle is **(A)** the Roman scissors handle with a rotating mechanism and a locking device. **(B)** The linear or coaxial handle allows a 360° rotation of the instrument in the surgeon's hand as well as a pincer grip of the instrument handle. *(Figure continues.)*

Typical Instruments

Operating instruments for laparoscopic surgery have several key features (Fig. 2-7). A typical instrument consists of a handle, locking mechanism, rotating mechanism, shaft, and finally the jaws of the instrument, which determine its functional characteristics.

Handle

A scissors-type handle (the Roman scissors handle) (Fig. 2-7A) with or without a locking ratchet is the most common form of instrument handle. This has been replaced in certain instruments (especially needle holders) with designs that allow a 360° rotation in the surgeon's hand and also the

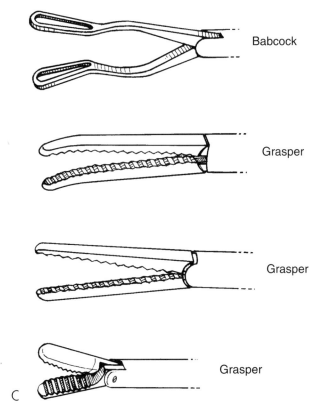

Babcock

Grasper

Grasper

Grasper

C

Fig. 2-7 *(Continued).* (**C–E**) Common jaw designs. (**C**) Graspers (note the wide jaws and dull tips). *(Figure continues.)*

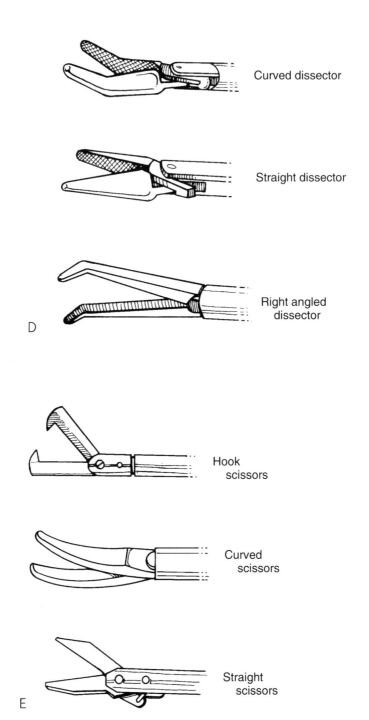

Curved dissector

Straight dissector

Right angled
dissector

D

Hook
scissors

Curved
scissors

Straight
scissors

E

Fig. 2-7 *(Continued).* **(D)** Dissectors (note the curved jaws and slender tips), and **(E)** scissors.

fine motor control associated with a pincer grip. (A pincer grip is the apposition of thumb to index finger or thumb to middle finger.) These handles are referred to as linear or coaxial handles (Fig. 2-7B). An example is the Castroviejo handle, shown in Figure 2-7B. A rotating mechanism (which allows the shaft to rotate relative to the handle) is often available with the Roman scissors handle instruments to allow a 360° rotation of the jaws of the instrument. This is a mechanical stepwise rotation that does not replace rotation of the instrument in the surgeon's hand but merely allows a repositioning of the jaws of the instrument relative to the handle. Some instruments are equipped with detachable handles to allow repositioning of the handle in awkward situations. Many instrument handles incorporate a locking mechanism to enable the surgeon to keep the jaws closed. This feature is especially useful for tissue graspers, where locking the jaws aids fixed retraction. Finally, a handle may incorporate a metal connector to allow transmission of electrical current during electrosurgical procedures.

Shaft

The shaft of an instrument should be long enough (approximately 30 cm) to reach the operative site while allowing half the length of the instrument to remain outside the abdomen. This "half in and half out" arrangement eliminates excessive or reduced movements of the tip of the instrument relative to the handle, caused by the lever and fulcrum effect of placing the instrument through a fixed point on the abdominal wall. The diameter of the shaft should be compatible with a standard cannula or reducer valve (usually 4.5, 5.5, 10, or 12 mm), to prohibit the escape of gas around the shaft. The surface of the shaft should be insulated to prevent the direct coupling of electric current during the use of monopolar electrosurgical devices (see below). The shaft should also be nonreflective because reflections into the camera compromise the image. A feature of the shaft of some instruments is the ability to articulate at approximately its distal third portion to provide an increased range of motion of the instrument. This is in some ways comparable to a wrist joint and may be useful by allowing the jaws of the instrument to approach the operative site from an angle that is more oblique than is possible with a rigid instrument.

Jaws

The jaws of an instrument determine its functional characteristics. An instrument may function as a grasper, dissector, or scissors (Figs. 2-7C–E). Almost all kinds of commonly available general surgical instruments are available in laparoscopic versions. Before discussing the unique features of some of the more common instruments, it is important to consider the cause and effect of the limited tactile feedback associated with these instruments.

Limited Tactile Feedback

A major limitation of laparoscopic instruments, especially graspers and dissectors, is their lack of tactile sensation compared with instruments used in open surgery. This reduced sensation is partly due to their length but also to the incorporation of more mechanical parts between the surgeon's hand and the tissue, compared with a similar instrument used in open surgery. Additional loss of tactile and force feedback (kinesthetic sensation) results from friction between the instrument and the cannula. The result is that the laparoscopic surgeon is less able to gauge the force exerted on the tissue; because the mechanical advantage is great, it is often possible to exert much greater forces than the surgeon would desire. The sites where this excessive force appears most likely to cause tissue damage are the base of the jaws (the portion closest to the instrument shaft) and the lateral edges of the instrument. This latter effect is the result of pivoting the instrument against a fixed point in the abdominal wall, which acts as a fulcrum, which can result in the surgeon exerting large lateral forces on the tissue as any movement with a medial to lateral or rotational component is performed. These risks need to be considered when using the instrument but also when choosing the instrument, so that a design that minimizes the risks is chosen, as discussed below.

Dissectors and Graspers

As the names imply, dissectors and graspers are used for dissecting and grasping tissue. The instrument should be selected with respect to its ability to perform a specific task while avoiding injury to the tissue being manipulated or adjacent tissues.

Design Features of Dissectors

Instruments with slightly curved slender jaws and relatively sharp tips are designed for dissection. This shape enables fine dissection as well as the ability to hold the edge of an organ or suture. The sharp tips of these dissecting instruments exert great force on tissues, with a subsequent risk of tearing if the instrument is used as a grasper, or risk of ischemic stricture and/or necrosis if the instrument is squeezed tightly for too long. Dissectors should not be used as graspers except briefly and under direct vision. Dissectors with jaws that have a right angle curvature (the right angled dissector; right angle Mixter) are also available (see Ch. 3).

Design Features of Graspers

Instruments with wider jaws and dull tips are usually called graspers. Sometimes laparoscopic graspers have specific names, such as Babcock, Alice, or Glassman clamps, in accordance with the similarity of the shape of the jaws to instruments used in open surgery. The shape of the jaws is, however, not identical to the instruments in open surgery. The jaws of laparoscopic instruments have usually been modified to reduce tissue trauma and to improve tissue handling.

Size of Jaws: Dissectors and Graspers

Jaw size is an important determinant of the characteristics of an instrument. Because the holding force of an instrument is determined by the pressure exerted by the surgeon and the surface area of the jaws, instruments for holding soft tissue usually have wide jaws. Care should be taken when grasping tissue with graspers or dissectors that have short jaws. Any instrument that grabs and holds the tissue for a prolonged time should have long and broad jaws. Although some manufacturers claim that jaws with deep grooves or a hole in the center make an instrument less traumatic by releasing the pressure at the grooves or holes, theoretically, a reduction in the contact surface makes the instrument more traumatic when the same grasping force is used.

Surface of Jaws

The direction of the grooves on the surface of the jaws of dissectors and graspers is also important. When an instrument is used to hold the tissue and retract it in the direction of the instrument axis, transverse grooves or serrations provide the maximal holding friction. When an instrument is expected to retract the tissue, such as intestine, at 90° to the instrument axis, longitudinal grooves provide the maximal holding friction. The shape and depth of the grooves determine the holding force and likelihood of tissue injury. Some graspers have teeth or claws at their tips. They are the most traumatic and generally are used only for holding tissue that is to be excised. The risk of tissue injury has lead manufacturers to design so-called atraumatic graspers, which limit the maximum force on the tissue when the jaws are closed and the handle is locked. Even they have the potential to cause serious injuries especially if contact with the tissue is unsupervised or prolonged. The tissue injury may occur, especially from the lateral aspect of the jaw from lateral forces, as discussed above. It is important, therefore, to examine the lateral edge of the jaws to assess the risk of tissue injury.

Single- and Double-Action Jaws

If only one jaw of an instrument opens while the other jaw is fixed to the shaft of the instrument, this is referred to as a *single-action-movement instrument*. Both jaws of double-action instruments move in equal and opposite directions.

Other Important Features

To reduce the risk of trauma from forces exerted at the base of the jaws (the portion closest to the instrument shaft), the jaws of some instruments (e.g., bowel clamp) are slightly separated at their base. In some instruments, hinges emerge from the shaft of the instrument when the jaws are opened. These instruments are not suitable for handling sutures or slings, because the fine material becomes tangled in the hinges. The ability to rotate the jaws is an important feature, except for the simplest maneuvers. It is also useful if the instrument has an attachment for connection to an electrosurgery unit. Some surgeons routinely connect their conventional laparoscopic instruments to electrocautery units to aid dissection, whereas others prefer to use a specific electrosurgical device, especially if it incorporates suction-irrigation.

Scissors

Shape of Jaws

Many shapes are available for laparoscopic scissors, which are named according to their similarity to instruments used in open surgery, such as Mayo, Metzenbaum, or Cooper scissors. Many disposable scissors have relatively broad jaws with a slight curvature. In addition, hook scissors are designed to cut tissue or a suture precisely. Microscissors used for microscopic procedures have also been modified for laparoscopic use. Metzenbaum scissors with their blunted tips are also useful for dissection. Scissors with sharp tips are good for piercing tissue. Curved blades, when seen on a two-dimensional

TV screen, provide the surgeon with an extra depth cue when compared with straight blades and may thus facilitate precise cutting.

As with graspers, other potentially useful features for scissors are rotatability, angulation, and connectability to the electrocautery unit. Some scissors open and close their jaws smoothly, while others are engineered so that a deliberate click is felt. In general, the latter type are less precise in their cutting ability. Both single- and double-action scissors are available. Double-action jaws are more difficult to manufacture and tend to be more expensive. Although the issue is ultimately one of personal preference, the fixed jaw of a single-action instrument may facilitate precise placement of the mobile jaw. The jaws of hook scissors and microscissors, which are the instruments used most often to create a small precise cut, are single action.

Instruments for placing sutures and tying knots are discussed in Chapter 4.

Retracting Instruments

Adequate exposure of the operative site depends on the appropriate use of gravity, retraction of adjacent organs, and traction and countertraction around the operative site (see Ch. 3 for further discussion). The surgeon's hand, gauze packs, and large retracting instruments used in open surgery cannot be used in laparoscopic surgery. The surgeon therefore depends on alternative forms of retraction (e.g., gravity), and in addition, some instruments have been specially designed as retractors for use during laparoscopic surgery (e.g., fan retractor). These retractors come in a variety of shapes and sizes. The basic requirements for retracting instruments are to hold an organ in position and to be atraumatic. To meet these requirements, retractors usually have wide finger(s) or prong(s) with some curvature and occasionally an option to change the angle of the jaws with respect to the shaft of the instrument. The wide surface of the fingers or prongs provides a broad area of contact to distribute the force on the organs.

Solid Organ Retractors

The essential feature of a retractor designed to retract solid organs, such as the liver, lung, or spleen, is to have a wide surface area in contact with the tissue. The most commonly used solid organ retractor is the fan retractor. These retractors have three to five prongs, which can be opened like an oriental fan (Fig. 2-8A). The prongs also have a slight curve at the tip, which unless used appropriately, may be harmful (see Ch. 3 for method of use). Fan retractors may have the capability of altering the angle between the prongs and the shaft and thus change the angle of retraction. An alternative design for solid organ retractors is a stiff balloon.

A one-finger retractor (Fig. 2-8B) that articulates between the finger and the shaft is also available and is commonly used to retract hollow tubular structures, such as the esophagus. The angle of the tip is changed by a simple joint between the tip and the shaft (the right angle retractor) or by using "memory metal," which is released from within the shaft and changes into its functional position.

Other Methods of Retraction

A Penrose drain, sling, or suture are all potentially useful for retraction in the same manner as in open surgery. The use of these materials is discussed in Chapter 3.

T-fasteners are useful for retracting or fixing hollow organs. T-fasteners are metal pieces attached to a nylon suture in a T shape (Fig. 2-8C). They look like the plastic devices that department stores use to attach price tags to clothing. A slotted needle is loaded with a T-fastener and inserted into the abdominal cavity percutaneously and then into the lumen of the hollow organ. A stylet within the bore of the needle is advanced, dislodging the metal piece (T-bar) into the lumen. The needle and stylet are then withdrawn, leaving the T-fastener in the lumen of the hollow organ. The wall of the hollow

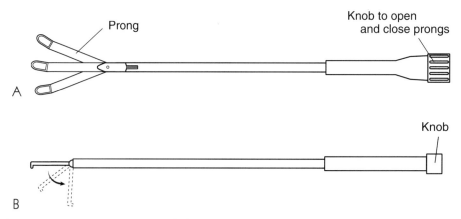

Fig. 2-8. Retracting instruments. **(A)** The fan retractor. Note the wide surface area of the prongs and the curvature on the tips. **(B)** The one-finger (esophageal) retractor. A simple joint allows articulation of the finger in one plane. (*Figure continues.*)

organ is then lifted by pulling the nylon suture(s) from outside the abdominal cavity. This principle could theoretically be used to retract other structures, such as the abdominal wall, or even parts of a solid organ, if appropriately sized devices become available. The use of this technique is further discussed in Chapter 3.

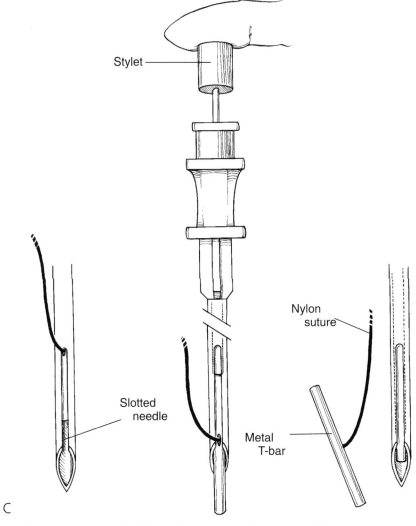

C

Fig. 2-8 (*Continued*). **(C)** A T-fastener, used to retract hollow structures.

Clip Appliers

A clip applier is a device used to apply clips to permanently close small structures, such as blood vessels, the cystic duct, and fallopian tubes, before dividing them. Both disposable and reusable instruments are available. Reusable clip appliers may be loaded with only one clip at a time, so the instrument must be withdrawn and reloaded for each clip, which adds appreciably to the operating time when many clips are used. Disposable clip appliers are provided with a rack of 20 clips, allowing faster sequential use of the instrument. The method of use of clip appliers is discussed in Chapter 3.

Laparoscopic clip appliers (Fig. 2-9A) usually have a trigger handle to deploy the clip and occasionally have a separate smaller trigger to load the clip before firing. The handle allows rotation of the shaft. The shaft fits through a 10-mm cannula and, in the disposable versions, contains a spring-loaded piston to advance the clips into the firing position.

The jaws of a clip applier are usually aligned in an almost straight line (15° to 20° angulation) with respect to the shaft of the instrument, although clip appliers with jaws at right angles to the shaft are also available. Clip appliers with straight jaws are useful when the clip applier approaches the operating site, making a large enough angle with the laparoscope so that the jaws can be clearly seen. The right-angle clip applier (Fig. 2-9B) is especially useful when the angle between the clip applier and the laparoscope is small.

The jaws of the clip applier are placed around the tissue to be ligated and when activated compress the clip into its closed position. This is done such that the tips of the clip meet first, so as not to extrude the tissue during closure. This is referred to as *distal closure* (see Fig. 3-11). Clips are available in three sizes: 6 mm (medium), 9 mm (medium/large) and 10 to 11 mm (large). This means that the clip applier itself has to be purchased in separate sizes.

An important feature of clip design consists of the serrations on the concave surface of the clip to reduce the likelihood of the clip slipping off the vessel. A factor that affects the choice of clip material is the likelihood of the patient undergoing subsequent radiologic examination. All metallic clips are radiopaque. Titanium clips have the slight advantage of not being magnetic and are not likely to interfere with a future magnetic resonance imaging scan. Titanium, unlike stainless steel, will not cause a starburst effect on a computed tomography (CT) scan. Only the image of the clip itself will be visible.

Clips have recently become available in absorbable materials such as polyglyconate. According to the manufacturers, absorbable clips provide an equal

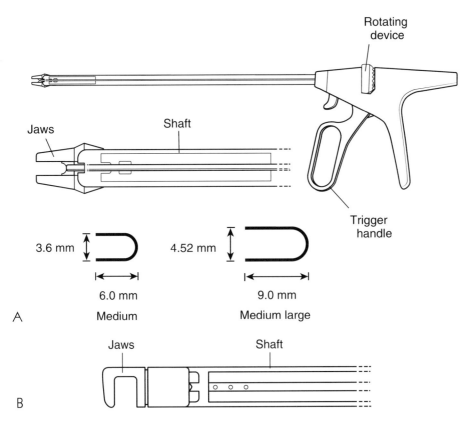

Fig. 2-9. (A) Laparoscopic clip applier. The jaw may be rotated to provide the optimal approach to the structure being ligated. **(B)** The right-angle clip applier. It is especially useful when the angle between the operating site and the clip applier is small.

or greater closing force on the tissue than titanium clips. Their disadvantage is that, because the material has no ductility, the clips need a locking mechanism, which makes them bulky compared with metal clips.

Stapling Devices

A staple, unlike a clip, pierces the tissue before the ends of the staple turn around to hold the structures together. A hernia stapler delivers single staples to approximate tissue edges or to attach prosthetic mesh to tissue. Stapling devices that deliver 4 to 6 rows of staples and divide the tissue between the middle two rows of staples are commonly referred to as *linear cutters or gastrointestinal anastomosis (GIA) devices*. Other staplers deliver three rows of staples without cutting the tissue and are used for closing a viscerotomy or lung (e.g., for treatment of pneumothorax). Circular staplers have also been adapted from open surgery for laparoscopic use. These different types of stapling devices are considered in the following sections.

Hernia Staplers

Hernia staplers (Fig. 2-10) were designed for use during laparoscopic inguinal hernia repair, although they have also been used with questionable appropriateness for other procedures, such as omental patch repair of a perforated peptic ulcer.[9] The use of hernia staplers for procedures other than laparoscopic hernia repair is subject to concern,[10] because the staples, designed to approximate a solid mesh, may cut through soft tissue. The hernia stapler deploys single staples to fix a single flat mobile structure (e.g., a hernia mesh) against another often less mobile structure (e.g., the abdominal wall). The handles and housing of hernia staplers are usually similar to those of a clip applier. Staples are made of titanium and come in two different widths, 9 and 11 mm. The staplers are available in both disposable and reusable versions.

Squeezing the trigger handle deploys a single staple, which pierces the two pieces of tissue and closes into either a D or B shape. The effect is similar to a single interrupted suture. For the disposable devices, the staples are available in cartridges, which may be reloaded a few times according to the manufacturer's specifications. The reusable staplers can deploy only a single staple at a time, so they must be withdrawn and reloaded between each firing.

In addition to a rotating device, some hernia staplers contain an articulating head activated by a sliding knob on the handle, which allows the surgeon

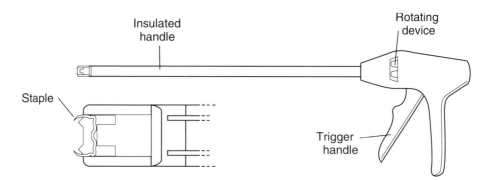

Fig. 2-10. Laparoscopic hernia stapler.

to address the tissue at different angles and place the staple perpendicular to the tissue. Although this feature may be useful in gaining more accurate tissue apposition, it also decreases the force that the surgeon can apply to the tissue.

Linear Cutter (GIA)

Linear cutter stapling devices (Fig. 2-11) are used in laparoscopic surgery to perform intestinal anastomoses, transect bowel, and transect large vascular structures (e.g., the mesoappendix) and blood vessels. Both disposable and reusable versions are available. A large pistol grip handle is squeezed to deploy the staples. In addition, there is usually a separate mechanism to open and close the jaws, as well as a safety lever to prevent accidental firing of the staples. In disposable stapling devices, releasing the safety catch and squeezing the handles together fires four or six rows of staples and then slides a blade within the jaws to divide the structure between the two middle rows. It is claimed that staples that close in a B shape compress the tissue hemostatically, while still allowing microvascular bundles to reach the cut edge of the tissue, thus reducing the likelihood of tissue necrosis at the site of transection or anastomosis.[11]

The staples are preloaded into cartridges. The cartridges for laparoscopic use are available in 30- and 60-mm lengths; it is important to note, however, that the cutting length of the linear cutter is less than the length of the cartridge. This cutting length is indicated by a black line on the stapling cartridge, and any structure beyond the line will not be divided. The other variable in staples is the staple depth, which affects the degree of compression of

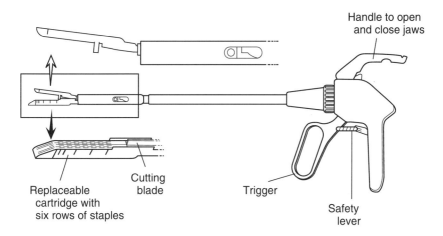

Fig. 2-11. Linear cutter.

opposing structures. A tight compression is required for blood vessels to prevent bleeding, while a looser compression is required for intestine, which is bulkier, to prevent ischemia of the stapled tissue. Staple depth (after closure) typically varies from 1 to 2 mm. The two major manufacturers (United States Surgical Corporation [USSC] and Ethicon) have color coded the cartridges to facilitate the selection of a cartridge for bowel (blue and green) or vascular (white) work. Tissue is typically compressed to 1 mm with the white cartridge, 1.5 mm with the blue cartridge, and 2 mm with the green cartridge. Disposable staplers may be reloaded with a new cartridge only a few times, as determined by the manufacturer.

Circular Staplers

Circular staplers (Fig. 2-12) have been adapted from open surgery for use during low-intestinal anastomoses (anterior resection) in laparoscopic surgery. As such, they are very similar to the devices used in open surgery to anastomose the rectum with the colon following a resection. This device consists of a long curved shaft, which is inserted rectally, and a head, which consists of two separate pieces that, when joined, perform the anastomosis. One part of the head, which stays attached to the shaft, consists of a circular plate through which the staples are fired and a circular blade, which emerges to cut the excess bowel inside the staples. Through the center of this circular plate, there is also a small trocar that pierces the rectal stump and docks with the other half of the head. The latter consists of a circular low-profile anvil, which is inserted into the proximal segment of bowel, and a hollow cylindric shaft that protrudes from the anvil and accepts the trocar stem from below. When the two pieces (the circular head with the piercing trocar, and the shaft of the low-profile anvil) are joined, they bring together the two segments of bowel, which can then be stapled together. Twisting a knob on the handle deploys the trocar and retracts it back after it has been joined with the anvil. A marker shows when the trocar has been unwound far enough. To join the trocar to the anvil, some manufacturers have incorporated a hollow shaft on the anvil (Ethicon), while others have made a solid shaft on the anvil and a hollow shaft of the side of the trocar (USSC). With this latter design, a suture is placed and tied through a hole at the apex of the trocar before inserting it into the rectum, so it can be easily removed by tugging on the suture once the trocar has pierced the bowel.

A window on the handle displays a marker to show when the edges of the bowel are apposed. This also allows the surgeon to choose an appropriate staple depth. A safety catch has to be released before deploying the stapling

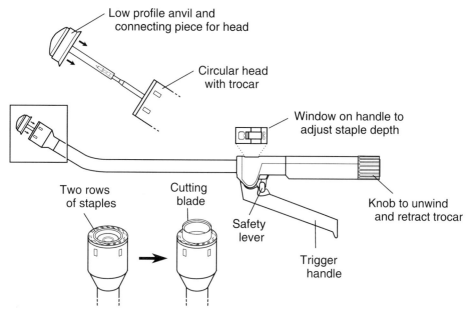

Fig. 2-12. Laparoscopic circular stapler.

device. Laparoscopic circular staplers are available in a range of diameters (21 to 33 mm). They have enabled laparoscopic low anterior resection. The difference between similar devices used for open surgery is mainly that the anvil designed for laparoscopic use is less bulky and is referred to as a *low-profile anvil.* This facilitates easy return of the proximal bowel into the abdominal cavity. (See Ch. 3 for method of use.) Manufacturers now make instruments that may be used for either laparoscopic or open procedures. These staplers are available only in single-use disposable versions, which adds $300 to $400 to the cost of the procedure.

Self-Retaining Arm

The self-retaining arm (mechanical assistant) is designed to fix a laparoscope or retractor in place. It is especially useful when repositioning is infrequent or when the surgeon operates without the aid of an assistant, as commonly occurs in private practice. Self-retaining arms are often cumbersome and may interfere with the movement of other instruments. Therefore, it is important to carefully plan its placement, especially when intraoperative radiographic examination is to be performed so that it does not interfere with the C-arm of the x-ray machine.

Self-Retaining Instrument Holder

A typical self-retaining instrument holder (Fig. 2-13A) has two metal components: a pole that is affixed to the operating table and a two-part arm that is attached to the laparoscope or retractor. The distal part of the arm has several joints to allow positioning of the laparoscope/retractor in any convenient configuration. The position of the arm is usually fixed by a series of mechanical screws or, in some models, an electrohydraulic switch.

Laparoscope Holder

Self-retaining arms that hold the laparoscope should ideally be equipped with a "zoom in" and "zoom out" feature, to allow the surgeon to rapidly and, easily change the perspective even during intricate parts of an operation, for example, suturing. As well as relieving the need for a cameraperson, they provide a steady picture. These semirigid holders are usually electrically controlled and may be activated by foot switches or hand switches. Repositioning of the laparoscope may require the surgeon to use his or her hands to redirect the scope and relock its position. Recently, computer-assisted instrument control has been used,[12] which measures the surgeon's head motions in real time and uses these motions to command a powered laparoscope positioner. The laparoscope holder has three degrees of freedom and has the advantage over the semirigid systems of not needing to be constantly repositioned (Fig. 2-13B).

Suction-Irrigation Devices

Suction-irrigation devices are used to keep the field clear of blood. They are of greater importance in minimally invasive surgery because even small amounts of blood may obscure the operative site and compromise exposure. Gauze packs, swabs, and sponges used in open surgery cannot be as conveniently used in laparoscopic surgery.

Suction-irrigation devices for laparoscopic surgery are often incorporated into dissecting and hemostatic tools such as electrocautery units (see Fig. 2-17, below). This helps to keep the operating site clean, facilitating fine dissection and the accurate identification and control of even small bleeding points. The suction element may also be used to evacuate the smoke produced during electrocautery.

Suction-irrigation devices are available in 5- and 10-mm diameters, both in disposable and reusable forms. In addition to the main opening at the end, the suction tip may have several small side holes along the distal shaft, which

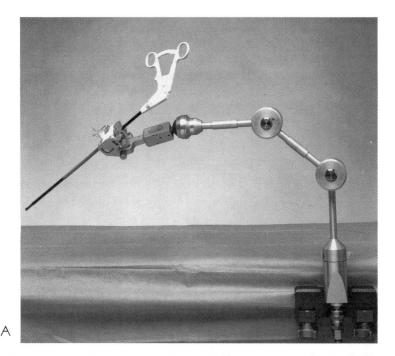

A

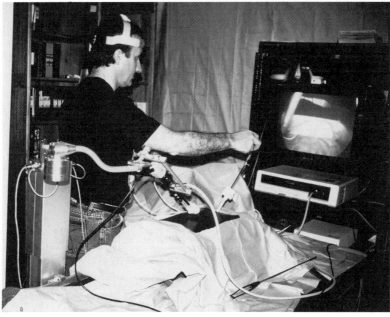

B

Fig. 2-13. (A) Self-retaining instrument holder. Note the hydraulic shoulder, elbow, and wrist joints, which allow the instrument to be placed in virtually any desirable config-uration. **(B)** Prototype of a computer-assisted laparoscope holder that measures the surgeon's head motions in real time and uses these motions to command a powered laparoscope positioner. (Courtesy of Dr. J. B. Petelin, University of Kansas School of Medicine.)

reduces the likelihood of the device clogging with fat or blood clot. The suction and irrigation may be controlled with a one-way stopcock or a trumpet valve. The latter is preferred because one can vary the intensity of suction and flow rate of the irrigating fluid.

The suction channel may be directly connected to the operating room vacuum-collection system. The irrigation channel is connected to a bag of irrigant fluid (typically, 5000 U of heparin in 1 L of normal saline) pressurized from 250 to 700 mmHg. A pressure bag may be placed around the irrigant bag and pumped up manually or with the aid of an electric compressor. A hydrostatic pressure of 300 mmHg is usually adequate for irrigating clots and tissue debris from the operative site. In hydraulic dissection, compressed gas is used to pressurize the irrigant up to 700 mmHg, and the irrigant can be used to dissect tissues, such as filmy adhesions or fatty tissues.

Tissue Retrieval

The laparoscopic surgeon often has to remove tissue, an organ, or other materials (e.g., sutures) from the abdomen. In some cases, this can be done just by pulling through a cannula. Often, however, the specimen is too large to fit through a cannula, and the surgeon must find an alternative method of retrieval. If this step can be left to the end of the procedure, the specimen may be retrieved through one of the cannula sites, which may necessitate a slight enlargement of the skin or musculofascial incision. Retrieval through a cannula site may also be performed before the end of the procedure, followed by an airtight closure of the defect, although this results in loss of a cannula site and a risk of subcutaneous emphysema if the closure is not airtight. In effect, this consists of a minilaparotomy, and in some cases (e.g., colectomy) the skin incision is made several centimeters wide to allow tissues to be brought outside the abdomen for an extracorporeal anastomosis. This is referred to as a laparoscopic-assisted procedure, rather than a complete laparoscopic operation. In the presence of malignancy or infection, it is desirable to avoid direct contact between the specimen and the wound, to theoretically reduce the risk of contaminating the edges of the incision.[13]

The simplest device for tissue retrieval is a sterile glove, plastic bag, or condom. All three have been used. Their disadvantage is that it may be difficult to insert the specimen inside and to keep it there during the extraction maneuver. Commercially available retrieval devices facilitate capture of the specimen and retention.

A typical example is shown in Figure 2-14. Resembling a butterfly trap, it may be inserted through a 5- or 10-mm cannula and unfolded using a grasper inserted through another cannula. The device consists of a long cylinder with a ring handle and a polyurethane pouch impervious to particles greater than 0.5 µm in diameter (similar to a condom). Typical dimensions for the pouch are 6 inches deep and 2.5 inches in diameter. Once inserted, a flexible metal ring holds the pouch open to allow the specimen to be inserted. Following capture, the pouch may be closed with a purse string by pulling a handle. This also detaches the pouch from the metal ring. The specimen may now be removed through the cannula site, usually at the end of the procedure. Similar bags are available that differ in their material and method of closure. Nylon bags are preferred when removing solid organs that need to be debulked within the bag. The mouth of the bags needs to be held open (triangulated) within the abdomen and, following insertion of the specimen, closed with a purse string tie on the bag (see Fig. 3-18).

In some instances, the specimen is too large (e.g., the spleen) to be removed intact through a cannula site. Alternatives to performing a minilaparotomy include removing the specimen through the fornix of the vagina or the lumen of the rectum (in colorectal cases). A large specimen may also be removed piecemeal after pulling the neck of the bag through the cannula site. Dejardin forceps or sponge forceps may be used in this method. Alternatively, commercially available tissue morcellators may be introduced into the specimen bag, which grind up the specimen to facilitate its removal. An obvious disadvantage of this method is that it may destroy valuable information for the pathologist.

Electrosurgery, Laser, and Ultrasound

Energy cannot be created or destroyed, but it can be converted. The application of electrosurgery, laser, and ultrasound in laparoscopic surgery depends

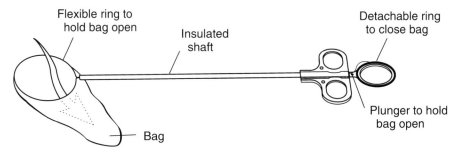

Fig. 2-14. Polyurethane tissue retrieval bag.

on converting these various forms of energy to heat. Many of the instruments are modifications of those used in open surgery. Nevertheless, some basic principles concerning the use of these forms of energy need to reemphasized, so that the instruments may be used safely and appropriately. In particular, a knowledge of the principles and risks of monopolar electrosurgery will help prevent iatrogenic injuries.

Principles and Risks of Electrosurgery

Monopolar Units: Ground Reference or Isolated Systems

If an electric current is passed through tissue, the resistance of the tissue causes some of the energy to be dissipated as heat. Most systems involve transfer of current between a metal instrument (the active electrode), which is in contact with the tissue, and the return of that current through a distant metal plate (the return, or dispersive, electrode) as the current seeks ground. This is referred to as a *monopolar system*. The dispersive electrode (ground pad) should have a surface area of 22 square inches, placed over muscular tissue, and coated with a conductive gel to enhance conductance. Older monopolar systems were known as *ground reference* systems, because current from the active electrode could return to ground through any site where the patient was grounded (e.g., the surgeon or any part of the patient that is in contact with metal). Although the current usually returned through the ground plate, there was also a risk that it could pass through an alternate site (typically a metal drip stand in contact with the patient's arm) and cause a burn (an alternate site burn). If one of these systems is used, it is important to ensure that the patient is isolated from any metal objects except the ground pad. We now use *isolated systems*, where the current can return only through the ground pad, which eliminates this risk. Another kind of injury with monopolar systems is pad site burn, which can occur when the ground pad is partially separated from the skin so that the current exits through an area smaller than the prescribed 22 square inches. An advance that prevents this injury is return electrode monitoring, which consists of an electronic system in the generator that continuously monitors conductance of the ground pad and automatically disables the instrument and sounds an alarm if conductance is inadequate (e.g., the pad is over adipose tissue or hair or is accidentally peeled off). During laparoscopic surgery, when the patient may be frequently turned and metal instruments may contact the patient's body, we recommend using a modern isolated system with return electrode monitoring.

Bipolar System

A bipolar system, in contrast, places the tissue between two electrodes, so the current passes from one electrode to the other through the intervening tissue. There is no need for current to pass through other tissues and thus no risk of the aforementioned injuries.

Tissue Effects of Electricity

Electric energy has three effects on living tissues. When an active electrode is in direct contact with tissue, the heat is dissipated into the tissue, and with time, desiccation necrosis occurs. This effect is often mistakenly termed coagulation. As the electrode is drawn away from the tissue, much of the heat is dissipated into the air, reducing the amount of desiccation but producing two remaining properties of electric current, namely, fulguration (coagulation) and vaporization (cutting). Coagulation is caused by sparks of high-voltage electricity passing through the tissue and is maximal when a low-current, high-voltage waveform is delivered (Fig. 2-15A). Cutting is maximal when high-current, low-voltage energy waveform is delivered, which (Fig. 2-15) causes a cushion of steam to develop between the electrode and the tissue. Tissue vaporization occurs from sparking across the steam gap. A blended waveform is a mixture of these two waveforms to deliver both cutting and coagulation. With a monopolar system, it is advisable to stroke the tissue gently with the electrosurgical instrument to maximize the cutting or coagulation and minimize desiccation. With a bipolar system, the tissue is usually pressed between the electrodes, so desiccation occurs regardless of the waveform used. Bipolar current is used principally for hemostasis. As tissue desiccation occurs from the bipolar current, the resistance of the tissue changes (Fig. 2-15B). An electrosurgical generator for bipolar current will maintain the waveform in the face of the changing tissue resistance. It is best, therefore, to use an electrosurgical unit dedicated to bipolar use when using bipolar electrodes.

Hazards of Laparoscopic Electrosurgery

Electrosurgery, although used by most surgeons, is not without risks, especially in laparoscopic surgery.[14,15] This is partly because of the decreased field

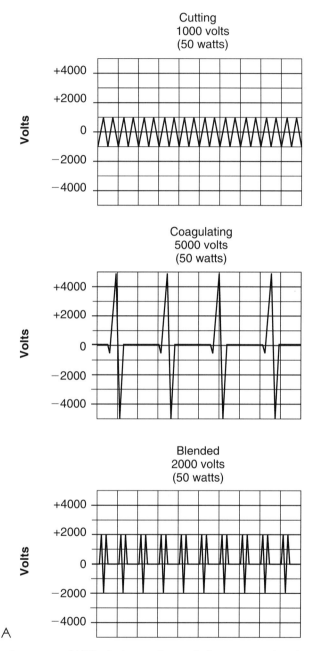

Fig. 2-15. Electrosurgery. **(A)** Typical waveforms during monopolar electrosurgery. *(Figure continues.)*

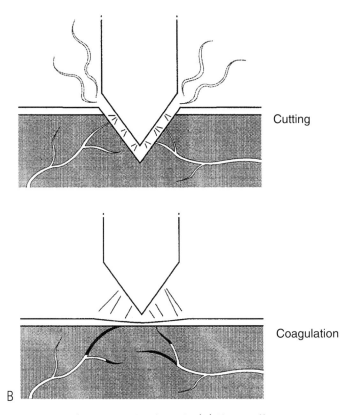

Cutting

Coagulation

B

Fig. 2-15 (*Continued*). **(B)** Tissue effects.

of view (see Ch. 3), which increases the likelihood of accidental injury and its concealment. The problem stems mainly from stray current, which may cause visceral injury during laparoscopic surgery in three ways:

1. *Insulation break.* A break in the insulation of an electrosurgical instrument allows current to flow from that point to any contacting tissue, where a thermal injury may occur. This highlights the importance of checking the instrument before use, by looking for cracks in the insulation. Greater vigilance is required with reusable instruments, because the insulation is more subject to damage with repeated handling.
2. *Direct coupling* (Fig. 2-16). The current may pass from the electrode to the laparoscope or another noninsulated metal instrument and cause a burn where this secondary electrode comes in contact with a viscus.

This is less likely to occur if the cannula through which the laparo-scope is inserted is made of metal, because the cannula can then disperse the current through the abdominal wall into the return electrode. This has lead some authors to recommend the use of all-metal cannulas during laparoscopic electrosurgery.[14,15]

3. *Capacitive coupling.* A capacitor is defined as two conductors separated by an insulator. Capacitors can store electric charge. During laparoscopic electrosurgery, the electrosurgical device behaves as one conductor, the surrounding metal cannula behaves as the other conductor, and the intervening intact insulating sleeve of the electrode behaves as the insulator. This arrangement can serve as a capacitor and accumulate electric charge if the electrode is activated before the tip is placed in contact with the tissue. As long as the metal cannula is in direct con-

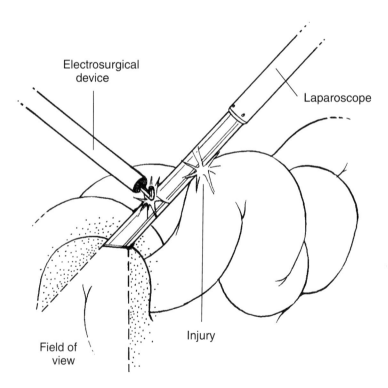

Electrosurgical
device

Laparoscope

Injury

Field of
view

Fig. 2-16. Unrecognized injury to bowel caused by direct coupling of the current from the monopolar instrument to the uninsulated laparoscope.

tact with the abdominal wall, the charge may escape safely to the return electrode. If a plastic fascial thread is used to anchor the metal cannula to the abdominal wall, however, the metal cannula is isolated from the abdominal wall, and the accumulated energy may discharge through a point of contact between the cannula and the intestine. Therefore, the arrangement of an electrosurgical device within a metal cannula that is anchored with a plastic sleeve is potentially hazardous. A useful rule of thumb is to always use metal sleeves with metal cannulas and plastic sleeves with plastic cannulas. Capacitive coupling can also occur between the electrode and another metal instrument. Capacitive coupling can be avoided by not activating the cautery until the tip is in contact with tissue, so the current has a route to reach ground and is not transferred into a capacitor.

A recognized hazardous situation is when electricity is applied to a relatively isolated tissue. For example, if monopolar current is applied to the completely dissected appendix or ovary, the only path that the current may follow to the return electrode is through an instrument or through the small area of tissue that still attaches the appendix or ovary. This situation may predispose to one of the three types of injury discussed above or may lead to an isolation burn — a concentration of energy in the small area of tissue that attaches, for example, the appendix to the caecum, creating a cecal burn.

Monopolar Electrosurgical Instruments

Electrosurgical instruments for use during laparoscopic electrosurgery have been invaluable in helping the surgeon to perform a hemostatic dissection. A typical monopolar device is shown in Figure 2-17. Both disposable and reusable instruments are available. The hand-held instrument is connected to an electrosurgical unit for the delivery of current in either cutting or coagulating mode. As stated earlier, if the electrode is immersed into the tissue, then regardless of the waveform, the primary action of the electrode on the tissue will be desiccation (tissue necrosis). The delivery of current may be initiated either by a foot switch, as in open surgery, or as is popular in laparoscopic procedures, by a rocker switch on the hand-held electrosurgical device (handset). Handsets that incorporate suction-irrigation devices also contain hand switches for these purposes. To avoid repeat sterilization, the handsets that incorporate suction-irrigation devices are only available as

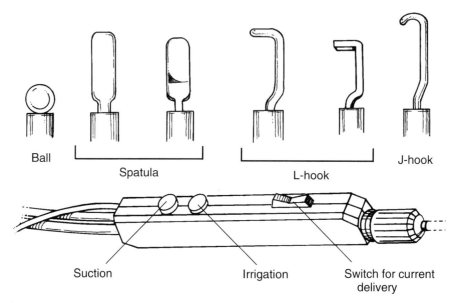

Fig. 2-17. Disposable monopolar electrosurgical device with built-in suction and irrigation.

disposable instruments. The design of the electrode tip determines the functional capabilities of the instrument, although there is considerable overlap between the function of different electrode configurations. Several common designs are shown in Figure 2-17.

When choosing between different manufacturers, the surgeon should appraise the cutting ability, coagulating ability, eschar build up, and ease of cleaning of the electrode. The build up of eschar and the ease of cleaning depend on the material used to coat the surface of the electrode.

Bipolar Instruments

Bipolar instruments (Fig. 2-18) may be disposable or reusable. Some regular disposable instruments are fitted with a connector for attachment to a bipolar system. An electrosurgical unit dedicated to a bipolar system is preferred, because this delivers the optimal waveform. As stated earlier, bipolar electrical energy is used for hemostasis. Bipolar instruments may be used to coagulate bleeding vessels (e.g., the use of bipolar graspers placed across a cut vessel) or the technology can be incorporated into mechanical cutting instruments. In the latter case, the jaws of bipolar scissors cut the tissue while cur-

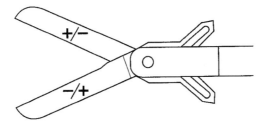

Fig. 2-18. Bipolar electrosurgery. The current passes only between the blades of the scissors, as each blade behaves as an electrode.

rent passes between the jaws to achieve hemostasis. The current has no direct cutting effect. Comparison between bipolar and monopolar scissors has shown that although both cut equally well, coagulation of tissue takes longer with bipolar scissors.[16]

Argon-Enhanced Electrosurgery

An alternative method of delivering electric current to the operating field is via a constant stream of argon gas, a method that avoids direct contact between the electrode and the tissue. The argon gas is delivered from within the tip of the electrode of a hand-held electrosurgical device that looks very similar to a conventional electrosurgical device. Argon is an inert, nonreactive noble gas, rapidly absorbed into the bloodstream and excreted by the lungs in exhaled air. It is heavier than air and easy to ionize. It is neither combustible nor does it support combustion. During argon-enhanced electrosurgery, an electrical current is used to ionize the argon gas, which is then delivered as a continuous stream of gas to a tissue. This results in a flow of electrons to the tissue. In this manner, electric energy may be delivered precisely to a tissue, without any direct contact between the electrode and the tissue. The characteristic of the electrosurgical waveform is maintained. The benefit of using argon gas to deliver the current is that the stream of gas may improve the ability to cut tissue by clearing smoke, water vapor, and blood away from the surgical site, thus improving visibility. In addition, the gas displaces oxygen from the tip of the electrode, which decreases eschar formation (carbonization) on the tissue. Argon beam cutting in open surgery has been reported to cause less blood loss compared with conventional electrosurgery.[17,18] Its use in laparoscopic surgery remains to be objectively assessed. The manufacturers caution that the delivery of argon gas should be restricted to 4 L/min to avoid

an excess rise in intra-abdominal pressure, which needs to be closely monitored. It is important to remember that the use of argon-enhanced electrosurgery is identical in principle to monopolar electrosurgery and thus possess-
es all the risks associated with monopolar current.

Laser (Light Amplification by the Stimulated Emission of Radiation)

The photon energy of light waves is converted to kinetic energy (heat) in
body tissues for cutting or coagulation. The impetus for the development of
this tool was the fear of injury from stray current in monopolar electrosurgery. It has been widely applied as such by gynecologic laparoscopists, but
after an initial surge of enthusiasm, most general surgeons have abandoned
lasers in favor of electrosurgery. The aim of this section is to review the basic
physics of lasers relevant to laparoscopic surgery as well as to discuss some
reasons for the differing usage by gynecologists and general surgeons.

Laser Physics

A laser is a monochromatic coherent beam of light. In other words, all the waves
of light in the beam are of the same wavelength, and they are in the same phase
in time and space. This coherence results in an additive effect of all the individual light waves. The particle responsible for the transmission of energy in a light
wave is a photon. The medical effect of a laser is due to the absorption of light by
the tissue and the conversion of the photon energy to kinetic energy (heat). The
major difference between this tissue reaction and the tissue reaction to electricity
lies in the concept of selective absorption. When light falls on a tissue, it may be
reflected, transmitted, scattered, or absorbed. Only absorbed light, however, is
converted to heat. The absorption of light by a tissue depends on the wavelength
of the light beam and the absorption characteristics of the tissue, that is, the
"color" of the tissue. For example, a green object is green because it reflects
green and absorbs other wavelengths of light within the visible spectrum. In
human tissues, a number of pigments absorb light and are known as chromophores. The major chromophores are hemoglobin, melanin, and bilirubin,
each of which absorbs light of a different wavelength. Water is also a chromophore, but it only absorbs ultraviolet and infrared wavelengths, which are not
in the visible spectrum. Black tissue (e.g., eschar) absorbs all wavelengths of
light. The theoretical advantage of lasers, therefore, is that its monochromatic

light beam selectively acts on tissues according to their pigment characteristics, cutting some while sparing others.

Laser Medium

The medium in which a laser beam is created, whether gas, liquid, or crystals, determines its wavelength. The most common media are shown in Table 2-1. The light generated by these lasers is selectively absorbed by different tissues. For example, carbon dioxide laser energy is highly absorbed by water; argon and KTP (potassium-titanyl-phosphate) lasers are highly absorbed by hemoglobin; and the Nd:YAG (neodymium:yttrium-aluminum-garnet) laser, which is poorly absorbed by water and hemoglobin, is moderately absorbed by melanin. The Nd:YAG laser penetrates deeply in tissue.

Delivery of Laser

Laser energy may be delivered to the tissues either as a free beam or as a contact tip.

The free laser beam may be delivered to the surgical site by a variety of laparoscopic catheter systems that may also incorporate suction-irrigation channels. The laser beam diverges 10° to 15° as it leaves the delivery catheter, so the power density decreases with distance from the catheter to the tissue (Fig. 2-19). The effect of the laser beam changes from cutting to coagulation as the delivery catheter is backed away from the tissue. The carbon dioxide laser, in contrast, creates a focused beam, similar to a beam of sunlight focused by a lens. Carbon dioxide lasers are not widely used in general surgery. The main risk with laser beams is accidental visceral injury due to past pointing of the beam. The laser energy may also be transmitted through

Table 2-1. Common Media Used to Generate Laser Beams

Medium	Wavelength ($\times 10^{-9}$ meters)
Carbon dioxide gas	10,000 (invisible)
Argon gas	488 (blue)
Nd:YAG[a] crystals	1,064 (infrared)
KTP[b] crystals	532 (green)

[a]Neodymium:yttrium-aluminum-garnet
[b]Potassium-titanyl-phosphate

the tissue being worked on and damage tissues elsewhere. For example, the bowel has been injured by using an Nd:YAG laser to excise a mucosal bladder tumor even though the bladder was not perforated.[19]

With a contact tip laser, the laser light is converted to heat by absorption of the energy at the tip of the fiber by a piece of metal, a sapphire crystal, or a cleaved quartz fiber. Thus, cutting at the tip is the result of heat, just as with electrocautery. The contact tip may be shaped to work as a knife or a coagulating instrument. Contact systems have the advantage of tactile feedback and the option of cutting with the side of the fiber. One problem is that the probe remains hot for 5 to 10 seconds after it is removed from the tissue, so the intestine can be burned if accidentally contacted.

Pulsing

Laser energy may be delivered continuously or as a series of short pulses. Continuous delivery allows heat to build up and to spread into the tissue to produce a larger lesion than intended. Pulsing may reduce this risk as the energy of one pulse is partly dissipated before the arrival of the next pulse. The damage, therefore, is more localized.

The Application of Lasers in Endoscopic Surgery

Lasers were in wide use by gynecologists by the time general surgeons became active in laparoscopic surgery. Indeed, in gynecologic practice, the laser has genuine advantages. Endometriomas, because they selectively absorb laser energy, can be dissected without damaging the adjacent tissue, for example,

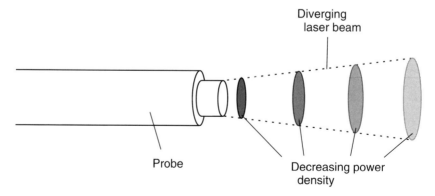

Fig. 2-19. Divergence of a laser beam.

bowel. Electrosurgery could be used, but laser avoids the risks of stray current. The influence of gynecologists was responsible for the initial embrace of laser technology by the pioneers in laparoscopic general surgery. In general surgery, however, there was no advantage, because there was no counterpart to the endometrioma. Compared with electrosurgery, lasers were found to be slower, more expensive, and less effective in controlling bleeding and also prone to complications. Not surprisingly, therefore, lasers are now rarely used by laparoscopic general surgeons.[20]

Ultrasound

Ultrasound results from a mechanical vibration and consequent sound wave at a frequency above the audible human range (i.e., greater than 18,000 cycles/s). Ultrasonic energy has been used diagnostically and therapeutically. Diagnostic tools have used ultrasonic sound waves while therapeutic devices depend on ultrasonic vibrations.

Diagnostic Ultrasound

A piezoelectric material is a nonconducting material that develops mechanical strain when placed in an electric field or, conversely, generates an electric signal if mechanically strained. An electric current makes piezoelectric crystals vibrate at high frequencies. If the crystal is in contact with the body, an ultrasonic wave is transmitted through the body and reflected at tissue interfaces. A second piezoelectric crystal is placed in the path of the reflected wave and the electronic signal generated used to indicate the placement of the tissues.

Laparoscopic Ultrasound Probes

Linear Scanning or Sector Scanning. Ultrasonic probes may scan a linear section of tissue by placing a large surface area of the probe in contact with the tissue and receiving an image of a linear cross-section of the tissue directly underneath the probe. The alternative method of scanning, sector scanning, whereby a small probe is used to scan a cone-shaped sector of tissue beneath the probe, is commonly used in laparoscopic ultrasound. Linear scanners, such as the one shown in Figure 2-20, have also been designed for laparoscopic use by placing the scanning surface of the probe at the side rather than the end of the probe.

Frequencies Used. The frequencies of ultrasound waves used for most purposes are 3.5, 5.0, 7.5, 10, and 12 MHz. The higher the frequency, the greater the resolution of the image obtained. Low-frequency probes are associated with the phenomenon of blackout, where the area immediately adjacent to the probe is not seen. The depth of tissue that may be scanned is smaller with the higher frequencies. In general, low-frequency probes (3 and 5 MHz) are suited to extracorporeal use, providing a low-resolution image but also deep penetration into the tissues. In contrast, high-frequency probes are usually chosen for intracorporeal use by laparoscopic surgeons, providing a high-resolution image of structures immediately below the probe but limited in their penetration of the tissue. As an example, a high-frequency laparoscopic ultrasound probe would be good for detecting tumors close to the surface of the liver, but the original low-frequency extracorporeal ultrasound may provide more information about a tumor deep in the liver.

The Use of Diagnostic Laparoscopic Ultrasound. The loss of tactile feedback in laparoscopic surgery has made the use of diagnostic ultrasound attractive.

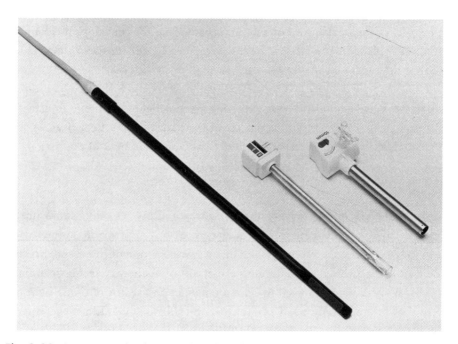

Fig. 2-20. Laparoscopic ultrasound probe. This probe fits through a 10-mm cannula. Note the scanning surface of the probe at the side of the tip (a linear scanner).

Used selectively, it can aid in the diagnosis of lesions or anatomic structures that the surgeon cannot see but in open surgery may have felt. Other than the diagnosis of hepatic lesions,[21] it has been advocated to search for common bile duct stones, gallbladder tumors, and identification of vascular structures before surgical dissection of tissues (e.g., liver, mesentery) where vessels are not easily seen. Although in this sense the ultrasound image compensates for the loss of feel, the image must be interpreted by the surgeon and is subject to artifacts unless used in ideal conditions (see below).

The ultrasound image should ideally be displayed on the same monitor as that from the laparoscope, so the surgeon may appreciate the structure being scanned. The probe may be placed in direct contact with the tissue, which works well for solid organs such as the liver. Alternatively, one can flood the field with bubble-free saline and place the probe just beneath the surface of the liquid. Ultrasound probes could also provide information about bowel mucosa adjacent to the probe. However, the mucosa-air interface on the luminal side of the surface being scanned reflects the ultrasonic waves, and the resulting artifact makes it impossible to interpret the image.

Several problems are associated with laparoscopic ultrasound. First, most surgeons are not trained to use the equipment and interpret the pictures. Training is an obvious prerequisite. The second problem is that access to the tissue is limited by the fixed position of the probe relative to the abdominal wall. Several manufacturers attempted to increase the potential area that can be scanned by designing probes with ultrasonic crystals either at their tip or at their side, which fit through a 10-mm port. Nevertheless, it is still difficult to use laparoscopic ultrasound unless the site to be examined is within the small surface area subtended by the cannula through which the probe is inserted. The high cost of ultrasound equipment can be spread over the many kinds of operations where it is useful. At present, ultrasound is routinely used in most hospitals to scan the liver during colectomy. The basic equipment is already on site. The only additional purchase necessary, therefore, are the special laparoscopic probes.

Therapeutic Ultrasound

When piezoelectric crystals or a magnetic device convert electric current to mechanical vibration, the motion can be amplified and coupled to a metal probe to transfer the energy to a tissue.

The use of therapeutic laparoscopic ultrasound makes use of two different properties that each depend on the frequency of ultrasonic vibration. In practice, the frequency of mechanical vibration of a piezoelectric crystal is inversely related to its amplitude. Therefore, at 23 to 24 KHz, the tissue effect is cavitation. At the higher frequency of 55.5 KHz, the lower amplitude oscillation of the probe gives a cutting effect.

Cavitation

The effect of mechanical vibration at 23 to 24 KHz is cavitation, which occurs as the pressure wave created by the surgical probe is transmitted through the tissue.[27] At a cellular level, this causes either an explosion of cells of high water content (adipose tissue, some tumors, the lens, etc.) or implosion of cells of very low water content (e.g., calcified tissue). The latter is similar to the effect of a hammer drill on a wall. Because tissues of moderate water content, especially collagen, do not absorb ultrasonic energy, some tissues, such as fat, are affected whereas others with much collagen, such as blood vessels, biliary tree, bowel, and muscle are not. This produces selective tissue fragmentation, which allows vessels to be skeletonized from within fatty structures. For example, the cystic artery and duct can be isolated from fat or edema within Calot's triangle. The tissue selectivity is a function of the amplitude of the vibration, as shown in Figure 2-21. Hence, tissue selectivity decreases as the amplitude of ultrasonic vibrations decreases.

An ultrasonic vibration may be delivered to the tissue as a continuous waveform or as a series of pulses. As with pulsing a laser beam, pulsing of an ultrasonic vibration allows the energy to be restricted to the point of contact of the surgical probe, which reduces lateral spread. Pulsing also slows the process of tissue removal.

Instrument Specification

A typical ultrasonic dissector consists of a hand-held surgical dissector, the acoustic vibrator, and a console. The console contains the generator apparatus and dials to control the amplitude of vibration, pulsing mode, and other functions, such as suction and irrigation.

The handpiece (Fig. 2-22) consists of a transducer, connecting body, and surgical tip. The transducer converts electric current to high-frequency mechanical vibration. The connecting piece couples the vibration to the surgical probe and amplifies the vibration. The surgical probe further amplifies the

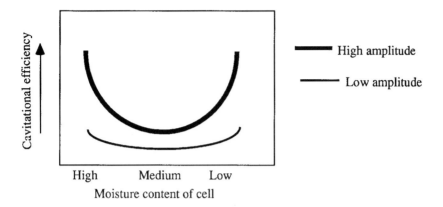

Fig. 2-21. Tissue selectivity of the ultrasonic dissector decreases at lower amplitudes.

vibration and transmits it via direct contact to the tissue. The surgical tip is made of hollow titanium. The handpiece may be refined to contain an aspiration-irrigation apparatus, so fragmented tissue is sprayed with saline and sucked into the probe. The transducer is surrounded by coils of coolant to prevent the instrument from getting too hot to hold.

Cutting

For ultrasonic cutting, a blade is made to oscillate at 55.5 KHz, a much higher frequency than used for cavitation devices, through a range of only 60 to 90 µm. At this frequency, the blade denatures collagen to form a coagulum, which seals small vessels.[22] This instrument can cauterize and cut simultaneously without the risks of electrosurgery.

Summary

Ultrasonic dissection allows the surgeon to fragment tissues selectively, which simplifies some otherwise difficult dissections. Whether this will be of value in laparoscopic surgery is unproved. The ultrasonic cavitating devices are already available in many operating rooms, because they are also used in open general surgery and neurosurgery. The laparoscopic handpieces are relatively expensive, but the cost can be spread over many operations. Ultrasonic cutting devices may be of value, especially when monopolar electrosurgery is risky (e.g., seromyotomy of the esophagus). Further assessment of this new technology is eagerly awaited.

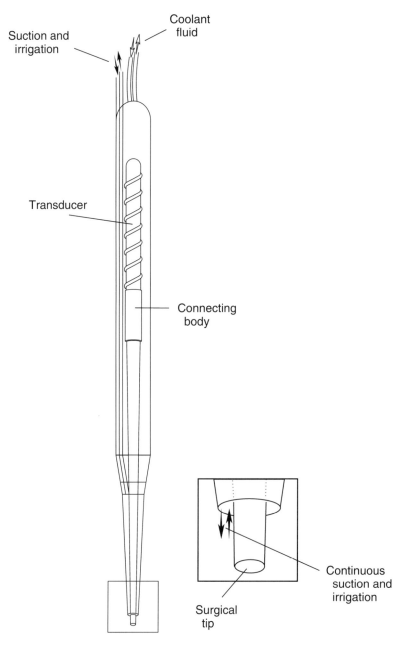

Fig. 2-22. Ultrasonic dissector with aspiration and irrigation channels.

Special Requirements for Thoracoscopic Surgery

Despite the long history of thoracoscopy, only since the early 1990s have surgeons widely adapted video endoscopic techniques to thoracic surgery. The list of conditions managed thoracoscopically is shown below. Although technical feasibility has been demonstrated, the appropriateness of managing some of these conditions thoracoscopically, especially malignant disease, is controversial. Estimates are that 20 to 30 percent of thoracic interventions will eventually be performed by minimally invasive methods.[24]

The thoracic cavity has different characteristics from the abdomen that have led to some important differences in instrumentation.

Diseases for Which Thoracoscopic Procedures Have Been Described

Pneumothorax
Bullous emphysema
Pleural effusion
Thoracic empyema
Hemothorax
Pleural tumors
Mediastinal tumors and lymphoma
Coin lesions
Chylothorax
Malignant pericardial effusion
Hyperhidrosis
Bronchial carcinoma

Imaging Equipment

The 0° rigid forward viewing scope is unsuitable for thoracoscopic surgery. This is because the wall of the thorax is rigid, and the surgeon often must work around corners to view the structures. The options are to use an angled rigid scope (e.g., a 30° scope) or a flexible fiber-optic scope. The drawback of the fiber-optic scopes is a lower resolution. The 30° scope is satisfactory for most uses, but there may be a greater role for flexible scopes compared with general surgery, especially if the quality of the image is improved.

Maintaining the Operating Space

The major differences between the thoracoscopic surgery and laparoscopic surgery are as follows: The thoracic cavity is rigid, so no insufflation is required; and the ribs restrict the size of the instruments to the width of the intercostal space.

Trocars and cannulas designed for use in thoracic surgery do not require valves as in laparoscopic surgery. Some manufacturers have produced oblong cannulas that fit the intercostal space. In fact, trocars and cannulas are not really necessary. Standard instruments can be inserted through small (1- to 2-cm) incisions in the chest wall.

Performing the Surgery

Instruments used by laparoscopic surgeons have been adapted with minor changes by thoracoscopic surgeons. Furthermore, as already mentioned, standard thoracotomy instruments may be used if trocars are avoided. Instruments of particular importance to thoracic surgeons are the endoscopic stapling devices. Current devices are the same as those used by laparoscopic surgeons, with two triple rows of staples. A staple depth of 3.5 mm (1.5 mm when compressed) is used for lung resection and 2.5 mm (1 mm when compressed) for use on vessels. The 30-mm linear cutter stapling device (i.e., 30-mm stapling cartridge) is most commonly used, simply because the 60-mm device has a diameter of 15 to 18 mm, which is often difficult to fit through the intercostal space in many patients. A major advantage of stapling devices for use in thoracoscopic surgery would be an articulating head for application of the stapler on the lung at awkward angles.[25] Such a device is under development. Another key instrument for thoracoscopic surgery is a lung retractor. Many such retractors are available. These fan retractors must be less traumatic than those used for liver retraction and also tend to have more fingers than liver retractors. It is also useful if the lung fan retractor can articulate. Similar scissors, graspers, and clip appliers to those used for laparoscopic surgery are used. Several suction devices are available for thoracoscopic use, but the avoidance of a cannula allows a standard Yankauer sucker to be conveniently used. Electrosurgery, laser, and ultrasound have been applied to thoracoscopic surgery in much the same way as for laparoscopic surgery.[26]

Summary

New instrument designs have made it technically possible to perform many minimally invasive procedures. Many of these instruments are changing, as it becomes clear that the unique problems in laparoscopic surgery cannot be overcome simply by adapting the instruments used in open surgery. Instruments, however, are not a substitute for training and skill. In addition to manual skills, the laparoscopic surgeon must appreciate the physics and engineering of the instruments to do the best job. Furthermore, the surgeon must be able to evaluate the claims of manufacturers. In a market where instruments are so similar, the choice between manufacturers often depends on service and the ability to upgrade when new versions appear.

References

1. Dorsey JH, Tabb CR: Mini laparoscopy and fiber optic lasers. Obstet Gynecol Clin North Am 18:613, 1991
2. Talamini MA, Gadacz TR: Laparoscopic equipment and instrumentation. p. 23. In Zucker K A (ed): Surgical Laparoscopy. 1st Ed. Quality Medical Publishing, St. Louis, MO, 1991
3. Monagle J, Bradfield S, Nottle P: Carbondioxide, temperature and laparoscopic cholecystectomy. Aust N Z J Surg 63:186, 1993
4. Reich H: Trocar shields seen as dangerous by some, others disagree. Laparoscopic Surg Update 2:49, 1994
4a. Bhoryrul S, Mori TM, Way LW: A safer trocar design for laparoscopic surgery. Results of a comparative study. Surg Endosc 9:227, 1995
5. Smith RS, Fry WR, Tsoi EKM et al: Gasless laparoscopy and conventional instruments. Arch Surg 128:1102, 1993
6. Idezuki Y: New technologies for laparoscopic cholecystectomy. An abdominal wall lifting device without pneumoperitoneum. Presented at the Saskatoon 1st International Symposium on Laparoscopic Surgery, Saskatoon, Canada, July 1992.
7. D'Arzi A, Geraghty JG, Williams NN et al: The pros and cons of laparoscopic cholecystectomy and extracorporeal shock wave lithotripsy in the management of gallstone disease. Ann R Coll Surg Engl 76:42, 1994

8. Baggish M: The most expensive hysterectomy, editorial. J Gynecol Surg September:57, 1992

9. Darzi A, Carey D, Menzies-Gow N, Monson JRT: Preliminary results of a laparoscopic repair of perforated duodenal ulcer. Surg Laparosc Endosc 3:161, 1993

10. Wyman A, Stuart RC: Laparoscopic omental patch repair of perforated duodenal ulcer with an automated stapler. Br J Surg 81:923, 1994

11. Steichen FM: Stapling Techniques, General Surgery. 3rd Ed. p. 3. United States Surgical Corp. Norwalk, CT, 1988.

12. Petelin JB, Chernoff WL: Computer assisted surgical instrument control. Presented at the symposium Medicine Meets Virtual Reality 2, San Diego, CA, January 1994.

13. Alexander RJ, Jacques BC, Mitchell KG: Laparoscopically assisted colectomy and wound recurrence. Lancet 341:249, 1993

14. Voyles CR, Tucker RD: Education and engineering solutions for potential problems with laparoscopic monopolar electrosurgery. Am J Surg 164:57, 1992

15. Odell RC: Laparoscopic electrosurgery. p. 33. In Hunter JC, Sackier JM (eds): Minimally Invasive Surgery. McGraw-Hill, New York, 1993

16. Edelman DS, Unger SW: Bipolar versus monopolar cautery scissors for laparoscopic cholecystectomy. A randomized prospective study. Presented at the SAGES Scientific Session and postgraduate course poster session, Nashville TN, April 1994.

17. Neven P, Sheperd JH, Wilkinson DJ: Radical vulvectomy using the argon enhanced electrosurgical pencil. Br J Obstet Gynaecol 100:789, 1993

18. Ward PH, Castro DJ, Ward S: A significant new contribution to head and neck surgery; the argon beam coagulator as an effective means of limiting blood loss. Arch Otolaryngol Head Neck Surg 116:921, 1989

19. Smith JA, Jr: Laser surgery for transitional cell carcinoma. Technique, advantages and limitations. Urol Clin North Am 19:473, 1992

20. Hunter JG: Laser or electrocautery for laparoscopic cholecystectomy. Am J Surg 161:345, 1991

21. Yamakawa K, Wagai T: Diagnosis of intra abdominal lesions by laparoscope. Ultrasonography through laparoscope. Jpn J Gastroenterol 55:741, 1963

22. Amaral JF: Laparoscopic application of an ultrasonically activated scalpel. Gastrointest Endosc Clin North Am 3:381, 1993

23. Meltzer RC, Hoenig DM, Chrostek CA, Amaral JF: The ultrasonically activated scalpel vs. electrosurgery for seromyotomy: acute and chronic studies in the pig. Presented to the Society of American Gastrointestinal Endoscopic Surgeons, Nashville TN, April 1994

24. Toomes H: Minimally invasive surgery in the thorax, editorial. Thorac Cardiovasc Surg 41:137, 1993
25. Allen MS, Trastek VF, Daly RC et al: Equipment for thoracoscopy. Ann Thorac Surg 56:620, 1993
26. Dowling RD, Wachs ME, Ferson PF, Landreneau RJ: Thoracoscopic Nd: YAG laser resection of a pulmonary metastasis. Cancer 70:1873, 1992
27. Hurst BS, Awoniyi CA, Stephens JK et al: Applications of the cavitron ultra-sonic surgical aspirator (CUSA) for gynecological laparoscopic surgery using the rabbit as an animal model. Fertil Steril 58:444, 1992

3

▶ Operative Techniques

T. Mori

S. Bhoyrul

L. W. Way

TISSUE DIVISION, EXCISION, AND APPROXIMATION ARE THE ESSENTIAL maneuvers in surgery. Although they are the same in laparoscopic surgery, limitations imposed by the imaging system and instrumentation require an additional set of skills for the surgery to be safe and efficient.[1–3]

Characteristics of Laparoscopic Operating Space

In open surgery, direct observation of the operating field and palpation of anatomic structures provide important visual and tactile information. The ability to perform any task is limited only by the surgeon's acquired motor skills. In laparoscopic surgery, the surgeon is handicapped by a limited view, impaired tactile feedback, and more awkward instruments.

Visual Perception in Laparoscopic Surgery

In laparoscopic surgery, the operative field is seen as a two-dimensional image acquired through a laparoscope. Depth perception is compromised, although stereoscopy is not the only source of depth cues. Shadowing, relative size of objects, movement of objects and instruments relative to each other, differential focusing of objects in the operating field, and the surgeon's memory of the position of an object in space all play a part.

Video Magnification

Magnification (usually $\times$ 2 to 4) of the viscera results in the surgeon's movements being amplified. This probably affects motor coordination. In the magnified operating field, distances between structures are more difficult to judge, and the amount of bleeding is exaggerated. The limited viewing angle of a laparoscope (approximately 76°) imposes another limitation. When a close-up view is needed, the narrow viewing angle makes the field of view restricted, so the surgeon is unaware of what takes place outside the visual field. The limited viewing angle also makes it difficult even to find the instrument when introducing it into the field unless the scope is withdrawn to get a wider perspective. The view of the operative site needs to be repeatedly adjusted, and this adds to operating time.

Manual Dexterity

In laparoscopic surgery, instruments pass through cannulas anchored in the abdominal wall level; thus, they are pivoted about this fixed point. The tip of the instrument moves in a direction opposite to the movement of the handle. The excursion of the tip differs from that of the handle, unless the instrument pivots exactly at its midpoint. These relationships complicate precise control of the instrument, especially for inexperienced laparoscopic surgeons. The set-up also restricts movement of the instrument to four degrees of freedom compared with six available to the instruments in open surgery (see Fig. 10-1).

Tactile Feedback

In laparoscopic surgery, tactile feedback consists only of what can be sensed through a long rigid instrument. Friction in the cannulas further reduces the kinesthetic sense. The handle of most instruments is configured as a Roman scissors design, which further reduces tactile sensation, especially when a locking mechanism is in use.

General Principles

Location of the Laparoscopic Surgeon

The surgeon should ideally be positioned facing the operating field and the monitor. The straight line on which the surgeon, operating site, and the monitor is located is referred to as the *axis of the operation* (Fig. 3-1A), and this positioning is referred to as a *coaxial set-up.*[4] A large (19-inch) high-resolution monitor should be used and placed close to the patient. Deviation from this arrangement will increase perceptual distortion to the surgeon and make the operation correspondingly more difficult. The importance of the coaxial set-up cannot be overemphasized. It may require the surgeon to stand between the patient's legs, for example during operations on the gastroesophageal junction.[5] In essence, the camera substitutes for the surgeon's eyes, so it should be in line with the surgeon's body and the monitor.

The location of the camera operator and assistant surgeon can also be analyzed. It is common practice for the camera operator to stand close to the surgeon and view the same monitor, while the assistant stands opposite to the surgeon and views an accessory monitor, also placed in line with the assistant's view of the operating field.[6] These positions work well as long as the assistant has a relatively passive role (e.g., fixed retraction of the gallbladder). The positioning must be reconsidered if the assistant is to be more active (as in a colon resection), because if the assistant is seeing a picture obtained from an axis opposite to his or her own, the movement of the assistant's instrument will

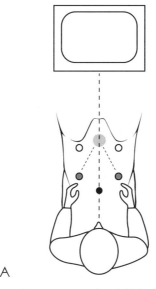

A

Fig. 3-1. **(A)** Coaxial set-up. The surgeon should ideally be positioned in a straight line with the operating field and the monitor. (*Figure continues.*)

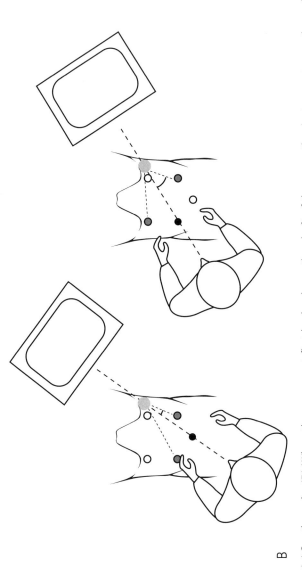

Fig. 3-1 (*Continued*). **(B)** When the camera at first looks down the shaft of the operating instruments, another axis is established by moving the laparoscope to a position where the angle with the axis of the instruments is larger.

B

appear to go opposite to the actual movement (a mirror image effect), making it difficult to guide instruments to the intended place.[7–8] In this situation, the surgeon and assistant may choose to stand close to each other, while the camera operator stands on the opposite side. Alternatively, the camera operator may stand between the patient's legs and close to the surgeon and assistant, or a laparoscope holder may be used and placed close to the surgeon.[9] Another way to decrease perceptual distortion is to use a single large monitor placed farther than usual from the operating site, which minimizes the angle of deviation from the axis that members of the surgical team view the field.

The coaxial alignment can vary during the procedure as the operating site changes. Ideally, the surgeon should change position to keep in the proper line. For example, the initial set-up for an operation on the gastroesophageal junction may be good for the esophageal dissection but not for dissecting the short gastric vessels; the change in operating site changes the axis. If the deviation becomes large enough, the camera may be looking down the shaft of the dissecting instrument, so the instrument eclipses the operating site (Fig. 3-1B). In this situation, the surgeon should establish another axis for viewing by moving the laparoscope or instrument to a position where the angle between the two is bigger.[10] Rarely this may require placement of an additional cannula if a satisfactory arrangement is not possible using the existing ports.[11]

Role of the Assistant and Camera Operator

The performance of the surgeon is partly determined by the skill of the camera operator and assistant, two roles often performed by less experienced persons. The camera operator must keep the horizontal plane properly oriented on screen and be able to use angled scopes so as to avoid visual distortion. Keeping the orientation horizontal is helped by features included in the design of the camera. There may be a red dot, cable angle, or box-shaped housing that indicates the correct declination. The best design provides clues by feel (camera shape) rather than by vision (red dot). The surface of fluid puddles within the abdomen also provides visual clues.

Handling of the camera is easy to understand. The quality of the job depends critically on the engagement of the person doing it. The direction of tilt of the objective lens for an angled scope is usually opposite to the position of the light cable attachment on the circumference of the scope. The camera operator should therefore steady the camera (horizon) with one hand and keep the light cable angled as desired with the other hand to get the best view

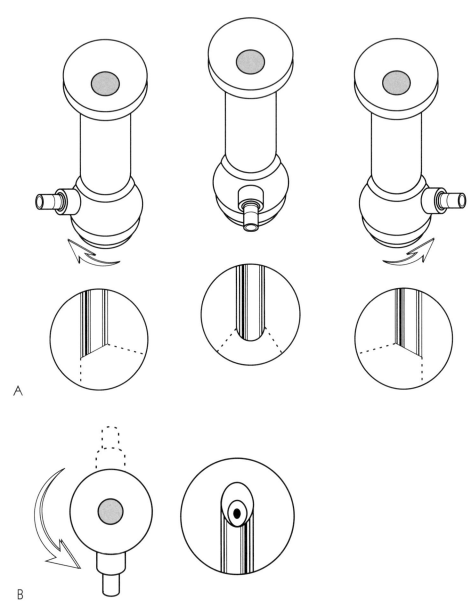

Fig. 3-2. Use of an angled laparoscope. **(A)** A different viewing angle is obtained by rotating the angled scope using the stem for orientation. A view from the right side is gained by placing the light cable in a 3 o'clock position and a view from the left side in a 9 o'clock position. **(B)** When the surgeon needs to look up at the anterior abdominal wall, the light cable is rotated to point downward.

of the field. As shown in Figure 3-2A, a different viewing angle is obtained by rotating the scope using the stem for orientation. For example, a view from the right side results from putting the light cable in a 3 o'clock position and a view from the left by putting it in a 9 o'clock position. When the surgeon wants to look up, the light cable should point downward (Fig. 3-2B).

The camera operator will often be called on to zoom in to provide a close-up image of a small field or zoom out to provide a wide view of a large field. In general, a panoramic view is preferred at the start to allow the surgeon to gain perspective and register the relationships between structures. When instruments are being exchanged or the surgeon is becoming reoriented, a wider field is also required. A tight view helps in performing detailed tasks, such as fine dissection, clipping, stapling, and insertion of a cholangio-catheter. In complex tasks, such as suturing and knot tying, frequent in-and-out moves with the scope are necessary.

The final role of the cameraperson is to maintain the image at the highest possible quality by keeping the objective lens clean and the point of the surgeon's interest in the center of the image. Thus, it is most helpful to have someone who can think like the surgeon handling the camera. A mechanical camera holder may be useful when changes in position are infrequent. Some of the mechanical holders allow the scope to zoom in and out in response to hand or foot switches or even the surgeon's head movements (see Ch. 2).

The role of the assistant is to maintain exposure and provide traction (exposure) on tissues where the surgeon is working. The assistant must know the steps in the procedure, follow the surgeon's instructions precisely, be patient, and be available for the whole operation. In general, the surgeon exposes the operating site and establishes the desired traction and counter-traction before handing the instruments to the assisting surgeon. The assisting surgeon then maintains their position until a change is required, which can be performed by the surgeon or the assistant if experienced.

When the surgeon operates with two hands, the assistant has a more passive role.

Display of Operating Field

Once the pneumoperitoneum is established, the surgeon must expose the operative site. There are three general methods of doing this: gravity, retraction of viscera, traction and countertraction. Failure to use any one of them leads to a suboptimal display and makes the job more difficult.

In general, the patient should be positioned with the target organ elevated so gravity pulls adjacent organs, such as the small bowel, omentum, or transverse colon, out of the way. The Trendelenburg position (feet up and head down) is used during procedures in the pelvis and lower abdomen, and the reverse-Trendelenburg position is used during procedures on the upper gastrointestinal (GI) tract and the biliary tree. The right lateral decubitus position is used for splenectomy. The right side is raised, and the head is dropped for appendectomy.[12,13] When the point of dissection changes during the operation (e.g., mobilizing the colon), the patient should be repositioned frequently to take advantage of gravity for exposure.[14,15] Elevation of the operating field also helps to avoid pooling of blood in the area. All these movements require the patients to be strapped down securely and an operating table that can be repositioned.

Retraction using retractors and graspers is vital. For operations on the abdominal esophagus and stomach, a retractor should be placed to lift the left lobe of the liver anteriorly and to the right.[16,17] A Babcock clamp may also be used to provide caudad retraction of the stomach. For laparoscopic mobilization of the colon, two atraumatic graspers may be used to hold the colon up and to display the mesocolon.[18] Penrose drains, vessel loops, or other slings are also useful retractors for bowel and other hollow organs.[19,20] Other specialized retractors (e.g., a right-angled retractor or lung retractor) are also useful in specific situations.

Traction and countertraction allow the surgeon to place the area of interest under tension. This results in greater precision and minimizes the chances of injuring underlying viscera, vessels, or other structures. It is important to place the traction and countertraction specifically on the tissue being dissected. The technique is as follows. First, if the target organ is attached to a fixed structure, then it may be grasped and pulled by a single forceps, while the immobile structure provides the countertraction. For example, during laparoscopic cholecystectomy, the gallbladder may be grasped and retracted laterally, while the immobile liver provides countertraction (Fig. 3-3A).[21,22] During laparoscopic appendectomy, the tip of the appendix is grasped, while the relatively immobile cecum provides countertraction.[23,24] The second method uses gravity as countertraction. When the target organ is attached to a mobile structure, such as the stomach to the short gastric vessels, exposure is achieved by lifting the gastrosplenic ligament anteriorly. Gravity holds the stomach down, providing the countertraction (Fig. 3-3B). The direction of traction must be away from gravity. If these methods are insufficient, the mobile structure may have to be fixed by a grasper or retractor. The third method is to use two graspers to pull the organ in opposite directions. This is a little more demanding and requires two instruments, but it is also more versatile and produces better results when the structures are mobile. An example is during seromyotomy of the stomach where two graspers are placed close to each other on the stomach to flatten out the area where the incision is to be made (Fig. 3-3C). This technique requires a skilled assistant.

Options in Laparoscopic Surgical Techniques: One Hand or Two?

The most common laparoscopic procedure performed by general surgeons is laparoscopic cholecystectomy. This is commonly done with the surgeon operating with one hand and relying on an assistant for exposure. The surgeon uses his or her dominant hand to manipulate a dissecting instrument while the assisting surgeon controls two other instruments. The nondominant hand of the operating surgeon can be placed at the base of the operating instrument to give it extra stability.[25] This technique is referred to as the *two-surgeons technique or one-handed surgery.*[26] Although relatively simple procedures, such as laparoscopic cholecystectomy, herniorrhaphy, and appendectomy, can be performed this way, it is not suited to more advanced procedures.

In open surgery, the surgeon works with both hands, one controlling the tissue and the other dissecting. Although instruments and perspective differ, the maneuvers that a laparoscopic surgeon must perform are similar. The advanced laparoscopic surgeon, therefore, must learn to work with both hands, as in open surgery. This is referred to as *two-handed surgery or the single-surgeon technique.*[27] Two-handed surgery is essential for the more technically demanding laparoscopic procedures. For these cases, the surgeon performs fine dissection, suturing, and knot tying, while the assistants handle retractors and forceps to maintain exposure.

Using Two Hands

When the surgeon operates with two hands, one instrument performs the surgical task (e.g., dissection and ligation) while the other assists by maintaining exposure and traction. Surgeons should hold the operating instrument with the dominant hand and the assisting instrument with the nondominant hand. As with open surgery, crossing of instruments is to be avoided. If the instruments cross, they clash with each other ("sword fighting"), and the jaws or shaft of the assisting instrument may eclipse the operating site. To avoid this, the surgeon may have to switch hands or switch ports. However, it may be

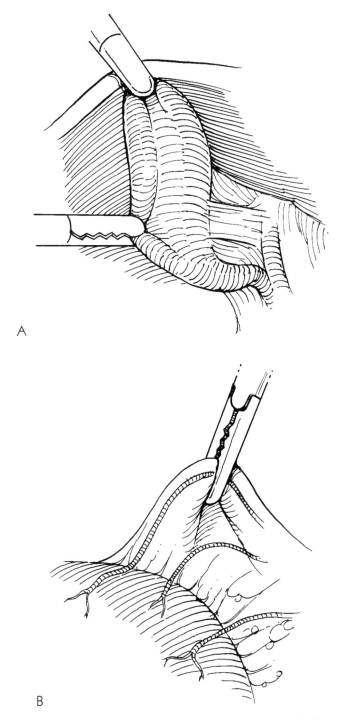

A

B

Fig. 3-3. Traction and countertraction. **(A)** If the target organ is attached to a fixed structure, it may be grasped and pulled while the immobile structure provides the countertraction. **(B)** When the target organ is attached to a mobile structure, such as the stomach to the short gastric vessels, exposure is achieved by lifting the gastrosplenic ligament anteriorly. Gravity holds the stomach down, providing the countertraction. (*Figure continues.*)

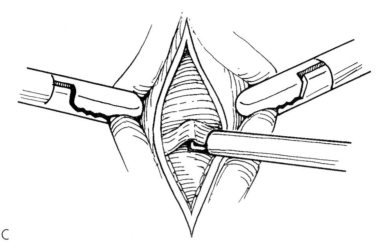

Fig. 3-3 (*Continued*). **(C)** Two graspers, grasping the organ relatively close to each other, are pulled in opposite directions, creating the tension between the instruments.

impractical to perform the demanding maneuvers with the nondominant hand. In this case, the surgeon may have to establish another exposure where those maneuvers can be executed by the dominant hand.

Gaining Access and Maintaining Operating Space

To create a working space, the abdomen is distended by insufflating gas (carbon dioxide) into the peritoneal cavity. Access for instruments and the laparoscope is created by inserting cannulas, which are also referred to as ports. These devices must have a valve or valves to keep the gas from escaping. The obturator within the cannula used to penetrate the abdominal wall is known as a trocar. The pneumoperitoneum can be established by a closed (blind) or open (Hasson) technique.

Principles of Port Siting

The positioning of cannulas for laparoscopic surgery determines the range of movement of an instrument relative to the operative site. Poor positioning can make the operation difficult or even impossible.

Cannulas allow passage of the laparoscope or instruments (scope port, operating ports, or assisting ports). The best sites for the cannulas depend on the relationship to the operative site. Placement is simple if the operative site is small, as with cholecystectomy or hernia repair. When the area is wider (e.g., colectomy), the strategy is more complex, but the same principles apply.

Cannula Site for the Scope (Scope Port)

The cannula for the laparoscope is most often placed in the midline. The most important factor is the distance from the operative site. When using the standard 0° scope, which measures about 35 cm long, a distance of 20 cm is appropriate. Thus, the cannula site for the scope is the point where a circle of 20-cm radius whose center is the operative site crosses the midline. This distance allows the surgeon to zoom in for difficult tasks, such as grasping a suture, and to zoom out for a wider perspective. Placing the scope port too close or too far compromises one or the other. When there is more than one area of interest, the position of the camera should be determined by the area in which the most technically demanding task (e.g., suturing) will be performed.

With an angled scope, the operative site can be viewed from different angles by rotating the scope, which allows the angled scope to be placed in a wider range of distances from the operative site than is appropriate for the 0° scope. Angled scopes, therefore, are particularly suitable for operations such as colon resection, where the area of interest varies widely. Proper use of angled scopes requires a more experienced camera operator. Of considerable help in deciding on cannula placement is a good knowledge of surface anatomy. It is common, for example, to see the scope port placed too caudad because the gastroesophageal junction is thought to be behind the xiphoid instead of the sternum.[28]

Port Sites for Instruments

Cannulas for Operating Instruments (Operating Ports)

At any moment during an operation, the surgeon may have up to two operating ports (right hand and left hand). The factors that determine where they should be placed are the distance from the operating site and the angle between their longitudinal axes and that of the scope port with respect to the point of dissection (Fig. 3-4A).

The distance from the ports to the operating site should be about half the length of the instruments (standard instruments are approximately 33 cm long) that will be used for the dissection, which gives the least distortion of movement at the tip from leverage at the fulcrum (the cannula). Because most laparoscopic instruments are 30 to 35 cm long, the operating cannulas should be about 15 cm from the operating site.

The operating cannula should form a 30° to 60° angle with the axis of the scope port (Fig. 3-4). If the angle is smaller, the operating instrument may eclipse the operative site. With a larger angle, depth perception is impaired,

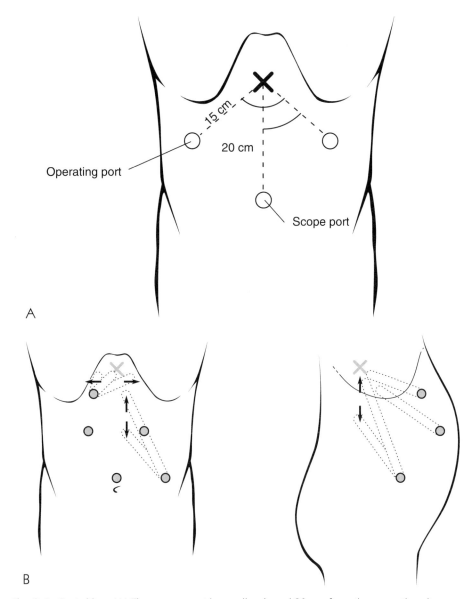

Fig. 3-4. Port siting. **(A)** The scope port is usually placed 20 cm from the operating site through the midline. The operating ports are placed approximately 15 cm from the operating site. The angle between the axis of the scope and operating port should be between 30° and 60°. The ideal angle between the axis of the two operating ports is 60° to 120°. **(B)** To avoid "sword fighting," the assisting ports should subtend an angle with adjacent trocars (either scope port or operating port) of 30° or more. If this is difficult to achieve, the assisting port should be placed much nearer the operative site than the operating ports, which gives a more vertical angle for the assisting instrument and decreases the likelihood of clashing with the more horizontally placed instrument. If the assisting instrument is to be used mainly for cephalad-caudad retraction of an organ, the assisting port may sometimes be placed further from the operating site than the operating ports. This results in the assisting instrument entering more horizontally, which minimizes sword fighting.

and fine movements become awkward. The ideal angle between the axis of two operating ports is 60° to 120°.

Cannulas for Assisting Instruments (Assisting Ports)

Assisting instruments (retractors and graspers that expose the operating field) are moved infrequently, so their locations do not have to be as precise as the operating ports. Important factors are the direction of the retraction and avoidance of sword fighting (instrument crossing). To avoid the latter, the assisting ports should subtend an angle with its adjacent trocars (either scope port or operating port) of 30° or more. If this is difficult to achieve, the assisting port should be placed much nearer the operative site than the operating ports. This gives a more vertical angle for the assisting instrument and decreases the likelihood of clashing with the more horizontally placed instrument (Fig. 3-4B). If the assisting instrument is to be used mainly for the cephalad-caudad retraction of an organ, the assisting port may sometimes be placed further from the operating site than the operating ports. This results in the assisting instrument entering more horizontally, which minimizes sword fighting.

The other factor is the direction of the retraction required. Placing a cannula close to the operating site optimizes medial to lateral retraction, while placing it further away allows better caudad-cephalad traction. When placing a cannula close to the operating field, there must be enough distance from the tip of the cannula for the jaws of the instrument to open.

When the dissection covers a wide area (e.g., during colectomy), port placement is more complex. Three solutions are possible. The ports may be placed so they can serve several areas of interest; more ports may be added; or the scope, operating instruments, and assisting instruments may be switched between the ports. The best solution depends on the individual case. In a Nissen fundoplication, the instruments can be switched so different ports are used by the surgeon for the esophageal dissection and division of the short gastric vessels. For a colectomy, an extra port is required to cover the entire field.

Closed Technique

Insertion of the Veress Needle

The closed technique for establishing a pneumoperitoneum involves percutaneous insertion of a Veress needle into the peritoneal cavity and insufflation with carbon dioxide. The needle is inserted through a small skin incision, usually at the site chosen for the camera port. This is most often in the midline above or below the umbilicus, except in the presence of a previous midline incision or portal hypertension. The open technique can be used in the midline, or anywhere else on the abdominal wall.[29] The skin incision should be long enough to accommodate the cannula. The umbilical crease is the most popular site for the incision, because the cosmetic results are best here and this is the thinnest spot on the abdominal wall.

When inserting the Veress needle, the surgeon can feel it pass through two distinct resistances: the fascia and the peritoneum. Some surgeons prefer to raise the abdominal wall with a pair of penetrating towel clamps or by hand on the belief that this fixes the abdominal fascia and thus helps the surgeon to feel these clicks. To avoid injury to the underlying bowel and large vessels, the needle should be angled 45° in relation to the abdominal wall and directed toward the pelvis.

Once the needle is in the abdominal cavity, its placement should be confirmed. First, it should be aspirated gently with a syringe to exclude accidental entry into blood vessels, bowel, or urinary bladder. Aspiration of blood is an indication to convert immediately to a laparotomy. If urine or bowel contents are aspirated, the needle should be removed and reinserted in the abdomen. After the laparoscope is in place, the bowel and bladder should be inspected, but injury to these organs is rarely significant from a needle stick.

From 3 to 5 ml of normal saline solution should then be injected through the needle. If the saline meets any resistance, the needle tip is probably in the abdominal musculature or the omentum. When the tip of the needle is free within the peritoneal cavity, the saline in the hub of the Veress needle will be sucked in, either by lifting the abdominal wall or by respiratory movements that result in a negative intra-abdominal pressure. If there is no saline in the hub, a drop of saline may be placed there to see whether it enters the abdomen (the Drop test).[30] The final confirmation of needle placement rests in direct pressure monitoring by the automatic insufflator connected to the needle. An initial pressure less than 7 mmHg would be expected, and anything higher suggests the needle is in the wrong spot.

Establish Pneumoperitoneum

Gas flow is initiated at a rate of about 1 to 2 L/min. If the tip of the insufflation needle is within the free peritoneal space, the initial pressure reading on the insufflator is typically about 5 mmHg, which represents little more than the resistance to gas flow through the needle. A higher initial pressure (greater than 7 mmHg) suggests the needle tip is in the abdominal wall, omentum, bowel, or mesentery (or the patient has not been completely paralyzed). In this case, insufflation should be stopped and the needle pulled back slowly, monitoring the pressure until it drops below 5 mmHg, at which point, gas flow can be resumed. If the pressure does not drop or if it rises quickly again, the needle should be removed and reinserted.

After about 1 L of gas has been instilled, if insufflation has proceeded normally, gas flow may be increased to 4 to 6 L/min. Some surgeons prefer to complete the entire insufflation at the initial slow rate on the belief that this lessens the chance of postoperative shoulder pain, but the validity of this notion has not been proved.[31]

The abdominal cavity should distend symmetrically during the insufflation. This may be verified by percussing all four quadrants. The insufflator should be set so gas is instilled until a maximum pressure of 14 to 15 mmHg is reached, at which point, gas flow will automatically stop. A higher pressure increases the risk of carbon dioxide gas embolus or deep venous thrombosis from disturbance of iliac venous flow. In an adult of average build, the amount of carbon dioxide required to establish the pneumoperitoneum at 14 to 15 mmHg is 4 to 6 L. When intra-abdominal pressure reaches this level, the insufflation needle is removed.

Trocar Insertion

Insertion of the Scope Cannula

Once the pneumoperitoneum is established, subcutaneous fat is bluntly separated to the linea alba using a Kelly clamp, a step intended to reduce the risk of bleeding from subcutaneous tissue as it is traversed by the trocar. Some surgeons prefer to make a stab incision into the linea alba to facilitate trocar passage, but this is not a common practice.

Before inserting the trocar, its parts should be checked to make sure they are functioning and properly assembled. When using a disposable trocar with a safety shield, push it against a towel or sponge to ensure that the safety shield conceals the tip of the trocar and locks into position immediately after the pressure is released. The trocar should then be re-armed and held in the surgeon's dominant hand. A self-retaining collar (fascial thread) should be on all cannulas except those used for fixed retraction. Grip the trocar and cannula firmly together until the cannula enters the abdominal cavity. It is critical to prevent overshoot of the trocar as it is being inserted, which is accomplished by fixing the wrist and elbow, using the shoulder to provide the force, while rotating the device. The instant that resistance is overcome, the force is stopped. Whether or not the automatic safety shield really offers much protection has not been convincingly demonstrated, and most experts are skeptical. Some surgeons prefer to lift the abdominal wall with a pair of piercing towel clips or by the nondominant hand to prevent it from being pushed posteriorly as the trocar is inserted. Whether this maneuver reduces injury to posterior structures has also not been demonstrated. Another trick is to lift the abdominal wall and instill additional gas until pressure reaches 20 to 25 mmHg. This is meant to increase abdominal wall tension and facilitate entry of the trocar. The safety of this method is yet to be established.[32]

When the trocar reaches the linea alba, it should be tilted 45° toward the pelvis to reduce the likelihood of injury to the underlying intestine and large vessels. Placing the patient in a 10° to 20° Trendelenburg position may allow bowel to fall away (Fig. 3-5). In an obese individual, the direction of insertion should be vertical, because the umbilicus is displaced caudally in these patients, and the shortest path to the peritoneal cavity should be chosen. The surgeon should pass the trocar slowly without loosening the grip on the device, which could result in deployment of the safety shield. Twisting the trocar may facilitate its passage. It is important not to wiggle the trocar back and forth, because this enlarges the path of insertion, which may result in a gas leak from between the cannula and abdominal wall.

When using a disposable trocar with a safety mechanism, the surgeon should feel and hear a click as soon as the peritoneal cavity is entered, which represents the safety shield snapping into place. If the safety shield accidentally closes before the abdominal wall has been completely traversed, the click is rarely heard, and resistance to insertion increases greatly. The trocar should be re-armed without taking out the cannula.

Once the click of a successful insertion is felt and the resistance drops, the surgeon should stop pushing. The cannula should then be inserted slowly 1 to 2 cm deeper and the trocar withdrawn from the cannula. As the trocar is withdrawn, a hissing noise may be heard if the stopcock on the device is open and gas escapes. The stopcock should be closed, and the cannula further advanced. The self-retaining collar should be screwed into the abdominal wall to anchor the cannula.

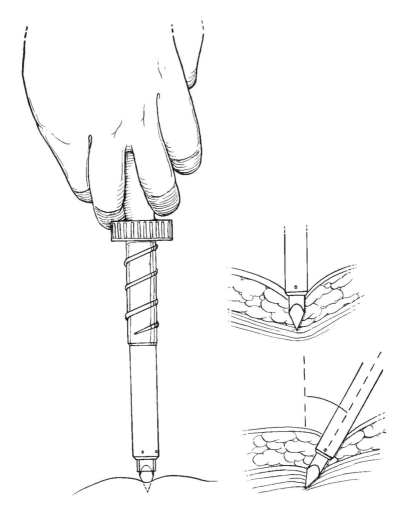

Fig. 3-5. Insertion of the scope cannula. As the trocar pierces the linea alba, it should be tilted 45° toward the pelvis to reduce the likelihood of injury to the underlying intestine and large vessels. Placing the patient in a 10° to 20° Trendelenburg position may allow bowel to fall away.

When using a reusable cannula, the stopcock for the insufflating channel *should be in its open position*. Entry into the abdominal cavity is indicated by loss of resistance as the trocar traverses the fascia and peritoneum and the onset of a hissing noise as gas escapes through the small bore of the insufflation channel. The trocar is then withdrawn, and the cannula is advanced further.

After connecting the gas line to the gas inlet valve on the cannula, the laparoscope is inserted through the cannula, and the abdominal cavity is inspected for injuries during the needle and trocar insertion.

Insertion of Additional Cannulas

Once the camera port is in place, other cannulas for operating and assisting instruments should be inserted under direct laparoscopic observation. The abdominal wall should be indented with a finger to select the proper site in relation to the operative site, adjacent viscera, and blood vessels in the abdominal wall. Care should be taken to avoid the path of superior and inferior epigastric arteries to the extent possible. If there are adhesions at the chosen site, the surgeon should either change the site or divide the adhesions with scissors introduced through another port.

Once a site is chosen for the cannula, the laparoscope can transilluminate the abdominal wall to check for blood vessels. This will be more effective if the light source is turned up and the room lights are dimmed. Another skin incision should be made and the assembled cannula inserted as before. The device should be aimed at the planned surgical site so the tract created through the abdominal wall is inclined in the correct direction. To do otherwise increases the force required to guide the instruments while using the port, especially in obese or well-muscled patients. Furthermore, frequent redirection of the cannula enlarges the defect, which may increase gas leakage around the cannula or result in its accidental dislodgment.

Under direct observation through the laparoscope, the trocar is slowly introduced through the skin incision with a twisting motion. The sharp tip of the trocar is clearly seen as it breaks through the peritoneum and enters the peritoneal cavity. The insertion should continue, taking care to avoid injury to the underlying viscera. If a self-retaining collar has been used, it is screwed into the abdominal wall. If there is reason to be concerned, the primary port site may be inspected by temporarily putting the laparoscope through one of the other ports, because injury caused by the first trocar may not be visible through the primary port. The laparoscope is then returned to the scope port, and additional trocars are placed according to plan.

It may be advantageous to insert assisting trocars before the operating ones. First, deciding on the best location for an operative port may be easier after setting up exposure with the fixed retraction. Second, inserting the operating ports may be easier and safer after a large organ, such as the liver, is retracted out of harm's way.

Open Laparoscopy (Hasson Technique)

The closed technique is popular because it is easier and faster and results in a good airtight seal around the cannula. Its main disadvantage is the risk of injury to the bowel or major blood vessels from the blind insertion of the Veress needle and first trocar (see Ch. 7 for further discussion). Open laparoscopy decreases this risk by placing the first port under direct vision by a minilaparotomy.[33,34] Either a conventional cannula or one of the many modifications of the Hasson cannula may be used. In practice, the Hasson technique is reserved by most surgeons for patients who have had previous abdominal operations or when it has not been possible to get a satisfactory position for the Veress needle.

After making the skin incision, which is usually just above or below the umbilicus, the subcutaneous tissues are separated by blunt dissection down to the linea alba. The linea alba is then grasped firmly with two Kocher clamps or Alice forceps and incised so as to enter the preperitoneal space. Care should be taken to minimize the dissection of the preperitoneal space, because this may cause the peritoneum to fall away from the fascia and make it difficult to incise. The peritoneum is then held up and incised. Entering the abdominal cavity is confirmed visually and digitally.

When using a Hasson cannula, a suture is placed on either side of the fascial defect. These two sutures may be tied together at the end of the operation to close the fascial defect, or newly placed sutures may be used. The peritoneum may or may not be included in these sutures. A Hasson cannula with a blunt obturator is then introduced into the abdominal cavity. The previously placed sutures are attached to the suture wings on the cannula with enough (strong) tension to plug the hole with the funnel-shaped obturator (Fig. 3-6).[35,36]

When using a standard trocar for a Hasson-like entry, a purse-string suture is placed around the fascial opening to secure the trocar and prevent gas leakage.[37] It may be difficult to expose the fascia to place the purse-string suture in obese individuals unless a large skin incision is made and the subcutaneous tissue dissected considerably. A disadvantage of a standard cannula for the Hasson technique is that it may slip out of position during the operation, because there is nothing to secure it in place.

A carbon dioxide gas line from the electronic insufflator is connected to the cannula. It is not necessary to set the insufflator initially at a low flow rate, because the position of the cannula in the abdominal cavity is certain.

Surgical Techniques

Although the perspective and instruments are different, maneuvers in laparoscopic surgery are not unlike those in open surgery. It still involves hemostatic dissection, excision, and approximation of tissue. The limitations in laparoscopic surgery require the surgeon to learn additional principles and techniques.

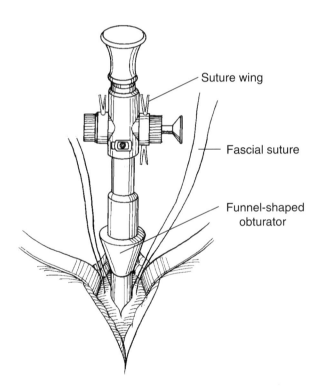

Fig. 3-6. Open laparoscopy. After placing a suture on either side of the fascial defect, a cannula with a blunt obturator is introduced into the abdominal cavity. These sutures are attached to the suture wings with enough tension to plug the hole with the funnel-shaped obturator.

Insertion and Extraction of Instruments

Insertion of Instruments

Inserting an instrument through a port is the first step in a laparoscopic procedure. The surgeon must first confirm that the instrument will actually fit through that port and that, if a reducer valve is needed, it is in place. Accidental tissue injury can occur, so the jaws of the instrument should be kept closed when inserting or removing it.

In their first 40 to 50 cases, laparoscopic surgeons should insert instruments under direct observation. The laparoscope should be withdrawn slightly and redirected to show the cannula through which the instrument is being inserted. When introducing an instrument, the port should be steadied with one hand and the instrument guided down the axis of the cannula. As the instrument is being inserted, the laparoscope should keep it in view until the operating site is reached.

Insertion of the instrument under direct observation is safe but time-consuming. Experienced surgeons eventually develop an ability to insert instruments without reorienting the scope and intuitively reach the operative field without injuring organs on the way. This should be done slowly to maximize tactile feedback in case viscera are encountered. Some surgeons prefer to introduce the instrument along the anterior abdominal wall until the estimated distance is reached and then the bring the tip of the instrument down. When using the blind insertion technique, the jaws of the instrument should be closed. When inserting instruments with curved jaws, the tips should point away from any organ that might be encountered.

Touch Confirmation

Once the instrument reaches the operating site, its position may be confirmed by touching something (touch confirmation). Touch confirmation allows the surgeon to memorize the position of the instrument in space relative to anatomic structures and other landmarks, which can be a valuable depth cue, especially early in the surgeon's experience.

Extraction of Instruments

Before extracting the instrument, the jaws should be closed because open jaws may result in accidental removal of the cannula. The flap valve of the cannula should be held open when extracting a hook cautery, suture needle, gauze, or anything else that might get caught in it.

Use of Instruments

The proper use of laparoscopic instruments will help avoid complications and shorten operating time. The instruments differ somewhat from those for open surgery, so they are used differently. The design of laparoscopic instruments is reviewed in Chapter 2. The aim of this section is to discuss their use.

Dissectors and Graspers

Although principles for tissue dissection and manipulation in laparoscopic surgery are the same as in open surgery, the limited perspective, the lever motion of long instruments, diminished tactile feedback, and limited access to the operating site call for additional precautions. In particular, the magnified view of the operating field requires the surgeon to make smaller and slower movements than in open surgery. Coarse, big movements are more likely to cause tissue injury and bleeding that interferes with the procedure.

The jaws of dissectors and graspers should not be opened until the tips almost touch the operating object. The tissue is then grasped under direct vision. Opening the jaws before the instrument is in sight may result in tissue injury. When performing blunt dissection, the instrument should be inserted into the tissue carefully with jaws closed; then the jaws should be opened slowly. It is safer to open the jaws parallel to the tissue plane at the start. Once a window is created, it may be more efficient to open the jaws at right angles to the tissue plane.

Laparoscopic graspers and dissectors may be used for blunt dissection with their jaws closed. Tissue can be teased away and pushed aside. Laparoscopic instruments may also be used as rod-like retractors when the jaws are closed, and the surgeon uses the shaft of the instrument to retract an organ away from the immediate field.

Care should be taken in grasping and retracting tissue. When applying a grasper, a generous amount of tissue should be grabbed to increase the contact area and to distribute the force. A small bite could slip out or tear. An equal distribution of the grasping force on the tissue within the jaws is also important. To achieve this, the direction of retraction should be considered, and excessive rotation of the instrument should be avoided. For example, when a grasper holds the wall of the stomach, the safest direction of retraction is along the axis of the instrument. When lateral retraction is needed, the instrument should not be rotated too much, because this exaggerates the force through one jaw and increases the potential for injury (Fig. 3-7A).

Injury can occur when an instrument is moved up or down (Fig. 3-7B). To decrease trauma during retraction, the grasper should be reapplied when a major change in direction is required. Graspers have the potential to cause injuries, and the site should be reexamined frequently and, if necessary, the instruments repositioned. A grasper should always be moved under direct vision.

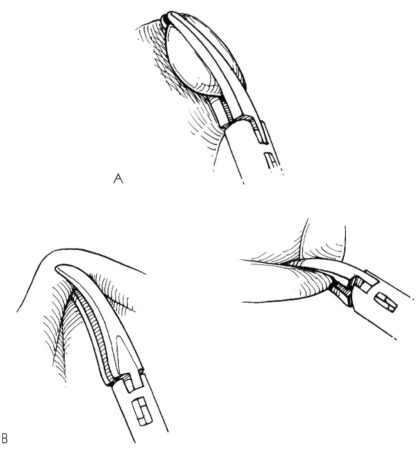

Fig. 3-7. Tissue injury by dissectors and graspers. (**A**) Excessive rotation of the graspers should be avoided because this exaggerates the force through the lower jaw and increases the potential for lateral injury from the jaws. (**B**) Injury can occur when an instrument is moved up or down.

Finally, some graspers have not been designed with blunt tips and round jaw edges, and they will be more prone to puncture soft tissues.

Scissors

The quality of the scissors is vital in laparoscopic surgery. The quality differs considerably between manufacturers, and we recommend that a careful comparison be made to find the best available.

As in open surgery, cutting is best performed when the scissors approach the structure at a right angle and the blades are applied perpendicular to the tissue. If the right angle approach is difficult, the tissue should be shifted around or another port chosen. Scissors with articulation or angulation mechanisms may be useful in some situations, but they are impractical for other than simple transection. When applying the scissors perpendicularly to the structure to be cut, the upper blade may eclipse the object. It is vital to see the tips of both blades before closing them. In this case, the jaws can be rotated slightly so the position of both tips can be seen, and then the rotation can be reversed before cutting.

Structures between the jaws of scissors sometimes slip out as the blades are closed, leading to an incomplete cut. This can be avoided by using a higher quality scissors or perhaps a hook scissors. The latter have blades shaped like a parrot's beak, so the tips come together before the rest of the blade (see Fig. 2-7E).

Microscissors may be useful to make a small hole in a vessel or duct to insert a cannula. The tips of microscissors are thin and sharp, so that they are easily damaged and rarely last very long. We recommend using a really good Metzenbaum scissors instead.

Scissors are usually designed so they can also deliver electrocautery through the blades. One risk of this practice is the relatively long electrically active section, which includes the blades and the unshielded hinge. This can result in accidental injury to tissues in contact with the uninsulated portion. One way to compensate for this is to open the blades when using cautery alone, which produces an angle between the tip and the shaft of the instrument. Metzenbaum scissors may also be used as a blunt dissector.

The use of bipolar scissors is discussed in the electrocautery section.

Retractors

Retractors come in a variety of shapes and sizes. A most important feature is a wide surface of contact to distribute the force to the tissue.

Fan and Right-Angle Retractors

When using a fan retractor, a broad contact surface and equally distributed forces are the keys to good exposure without damaging tissues. Ideally, the direction of retraction should be perpendicular to the surface of the blades. To achieve this, the cannula through which the retractors are inserted should be appropriately sited. Fan retractors with an articulating shaft may occasionally be useful when it is difficult to site the port properly for a standard straight retractor.

When introducing a fan retractor into the abdominal cavity, the prongs should be kept closed until the final position is reached. To guide placement of the retractor, a second instrument may be useful to lift the edge of the organ (e.g., liver) being retracted.

Force is often greatest at the tips of a fan retractor. For example, when retracting the liver, the tips of the retractor are most likely to puncture the capsule. To avoid this, the fan retractor should be inserted deep enough to distribute the forces over the whole surface of the blade, not just the tip. The prongs of fan retractors sometimes have curved tips, which should be placed to face *away* from the surface of the liver but *toward* the surface of bowel (Fig. 3-8A).

One-finger retractors are relatively safe and effective. Retraction of the organ is best achieved when the finger is inserted from the same side of direction of traction under direct laparoscopic observation (Fig. 3-8B).

T-Fasteners

A T-fastener is a 1-cm metal rod attached at its midpoint to a nylon suture in a T shape,[38] which can be used as a retractor for hollow organs (see Fig. 2-8C).

A slotted needle is loaded with the bar and inserted into the abdominal cavity percutaneously under laparoscopic guidance. The needle is introduced into the lumen of a hollow organ, and the T-bar dislodged into the lumen by a stylet passed down the hollow of the needle. To lessen the chance of penetrating the back wall, the lumen should be insufflated with carbon dioxide or air, if possible. Before inserting the needle into the lumen of the gut, the intra-abdominal pressure may be decreased to 5 mmHg or less, which allows the gas in the gut to expand the lumen and the abdominal wall to come closer to the gut wall. The needle and stylet are then withdrawn, leaving the T-bar in the lumen (Fig. 3-9).[39] The gut wall is then retracted by pulling the nylon suture from outside the abdominal cavity.

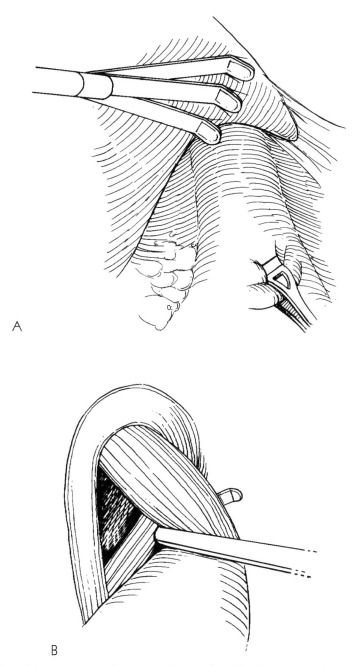

A

B

Fig. 3-8. (**A**) Fan retractor. When retracting the liver, the fan retractor is inserted deep enough to distribute the forces over the whole surface of the blade. The curved tips of the blade should be placed to face away from the surface of the liver. (**B**) One-finger retractor. Retraction of the organ is best achieved when the finger is inserted from the same side of direction of traction.

During a partial resection for gastric or colonic lesions, T-fasteners may be placed around or through the lesion under the guidance of the endoscope. The wall is then retracted by pulling on the T-fasteners, and a linear anastomoser is applied and fired below the lesion, partially excising the wall.

T-fasteners are also used to anchor the wall of the stomach, small intestine, or colon to the anterior abdominal wall for enterostomies.[40] Four T-fasteners are placed in a diamond shape, and a feeding tube or catheter is inserted in the middle. After inserting the tube, the T-fasteners are pulled to appose the

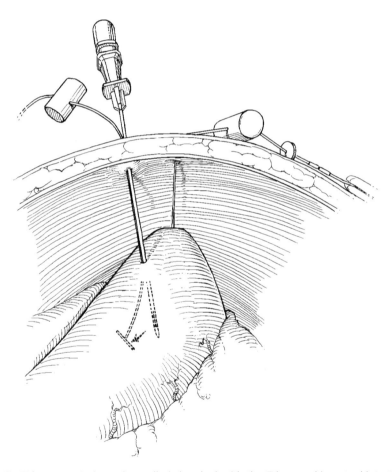

Fig. 3-9. T-fastener. A slotted needle is loaded with the T-bar and inserted into the abdominal cavity percutaneously and then into the lumen of the hollow organ. The T-bar is dislodged into the lumen by a stylet passed down the hollow of the needle. The suture is then pulled to retract the organ.

enterostomy site to the abdominal wall, and the nylon sutures are then secured outside by crimping metal hubs.

Other Methods of Retraction

Penrose drains, slings, and sutures are sometimes useful for retraction. The esophagus, for example, can be retracted by a Penrose drain encircling the esophagogastric junction (Fig. 3-10A). For laparoscopic mobilization of the colon, a suture may be inserted through the abdominal wall and mesocolon and then brought out through the abdominal wall again. This holds the colon anteriorly, exposing the mesocolon.

Sutures can also be used for retraction by applying a pretied loop to an organ. For example, during appendectomy, a Roeder loop may be applied to the tip of the appendix and held by a grasper, which helps display the mesoappendix (Fig. 3-10B).

These methods tend to be more flexible and less traumatic than conventional tissue retractors.

Clip Appliers

Clips can be used to occlude vessels or tubular structures of small caliber, such as the cystic duct or Fallopian tube. Clips are good for these tasks, because other means, such as ligating with sutures are more difficult.

With a reusable single-fire clip applier, extra care is needed to avoid dislodging the clip as the instrument is inserted. Accidental partial compression of the handle predisposes to dislodgment. Disposable multifire clip appliers are loaded by a separate trigger or by the first reaction from squeezing the handle. In some versions, the handle cannot be closed when the jaws are empty.

The structure to be occluded should be dissected circumferentially from the surrounding tissue, otherwise important adjacent structures (e.g., common hepatic duct while clipping the cystic duct) might be involved in the clip. Intervening soft tissue in the clip may also make occlusion incomplete. Once a complete window is created around the structure, it should be extended 1.5 to 2.0 cm along the longitudinal axis. The clip applier is inserted so it approaches its target at an angle of 45° to 90° relative to the laparoscope, which permits viewing the clip loaded in place. With this arrangement, the entire procedure can be executed under direct view. If the clip applier approaches the structure end on, the jaws of a standard straight arm clip applier may be eclipsed by its shaft or by the structure to be clipped. In this

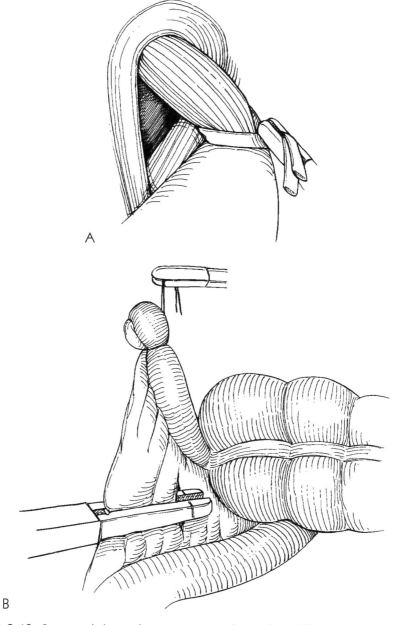

Fig. 3-10. Penrose drains and sutures as retracting tools. (**A**) The esophagus can be retracted by a Penrose drain encircling the esophagogastric junction. (**B**) During appendectomy, a Roeder loop may be applied to the tip of the appendix and held by a grasper, which helps display the mesoappendix.

situation, a right-angle (side biting) clip applier may be better because clips can be applied from the side. More often, the problem is solved by gaining a different perspective with a 30° scope.

When passing the clip applier across tissue, both jaws must be visible. When the lower jaw is eclipsed by the upper jaw, the shaft should be rotated to permit a view of the lower jaw (Fig. 3-11A). Once placement is good, the jaws are re-rotated to the optimal position. The handles are squeezed slowly to the half-closed position, watching the tips of the clip come together. In the half-compressed configuration (teardrop shape), the clip can be slid up or down along the structure, which allows the clip to be placed precisely (Fig. 3-11B).

Once the jaws are positioned, the handles are squeezed firmly, compressing and flattening the clip to occlude the lumen of the structure. Then the grip is relaxed, and the device is withdrawn. Typically, four clips are used on small blood vessels and the cystic duct, and five clips on larger vessels.

Before dividing the structure, the surgeon should confirm that the clips span its width and that the tips have come together free of tissue. Usually, two clips should be on each side.

When unexpected bleeding occurs, it may be necessary to control it with clips. This can be tricky. The technique is discussed later.

Stapling Devices

Hernia Stapler

Hernia staplers are available in both disposable and reusable versions. The reusable devices are single fire and must be withdrawn and reloaded after each use. They are better suited to placing staples on firm tissue, such as Cooper's ligament, because they have a metal shaft. When a series of staples is required, the disposable multifire stapler reduces operating time.

Hernia staplers require an 11-mm or larger cannula. Stapling is best performed when the stapler approaches the operating site perpendicularly and forms an angle with the laparoscope of approximately 60°. During laparoscopic hernia repair, the stapler is inserted from the same side as the repair. Articulation of the shaft sometimes facilitates placing the staples when it is difficult to obtain a perpendicular approach to the operating site.

With a reusable single-fire stapler, care should be taken to avoid dislodging the staple as the instrument is inserted. Partially squeezed handles are the most common cause of dislodgment.

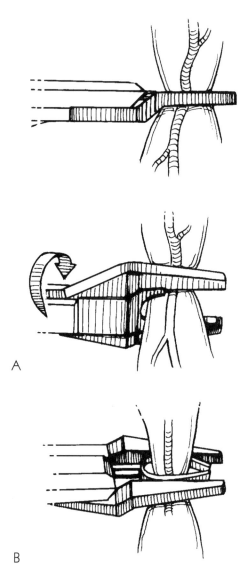

Fig. 3-11. Applying clips. (**A**) When passing the clip applier across the tissue, both jaws must be visible. When the lower jaw is eclipsed by the upper jaw, the shaft should be rotated to see the lower jaw. (**B**) A half-compressed clip (teardrop shape) can be slid up or down along the structure, which allows the clip to be placed precisely.

When approximating tissue edges, they should be brought close to each other before placing staples, which can be accomplished by two methods. The first method is "tip-to-tip" approximation, in which a grasper from the right grabs the right side of the tissue edge, and another grasper from the left grabs the opposite edge. Both edges are approximated by placing the graspers tip to tip (Fig. 3-12A). The alternative method is the "X arrangement," in which a grasper from the right grabs the left side of the tissue edge, while another grasper from the left grabs the right edge 2 to 3 cm away from the first grasper. Both graspers are then pulled so the tissue flaps overlap for 1 to 1.5 cm. The tissue edges are approximated at the point where the edges cross, forming an X shape (Fig. 3-12B).

The jaws of the stapler are rotated so the staple is placed at right angles to the line of tissue closure. The jaws are placed so the same amount of tissue is included in the staple on either side. Once position is satisfactory, the jaws are pushed against the tissue, and the handles are squeezed slowly and firmly; the surgeon should watch that the ends of the staple exit the jaws straight and parallel to each other as they enter the tissue. As the handles are further squeezed, the staple is molded into a D or B shape, as it apposes both edges. Then the grip is relaxed.

Once the edges are apposed with the first staple, two instruments are no longer required for approximation, because the staple maintains the position. The tissue edges can now be approximated by holding them together with a grasper or by holding one side and pushing it against the other.

A third method of tissue approximation with the hernia stapler is to squeeze the handles enough to make the tips of the staple partially exit from the jaws. One tip is pushed into the tissue, the opposite edge is pulled into position, and then the staple is fired (Fig. 3-12C). This technique is useful when only one grasper can be used.

As the name indicates, hernia staplers are most commonly used to fix a hernia mesh in place and to reperitonealize in laparoscopic hernia repair. When fixing the mesh, gentle counterpressure with a hand against the abdominal wall facilitates placing all but the Cooper's ligament staples.

Linear Cutter (Gastrointestinal Anastomoser)

The factors to be considered in selecting a linear cutter are the length of the jaws and the staple depth. They are available in 30- or 60-mm staple line

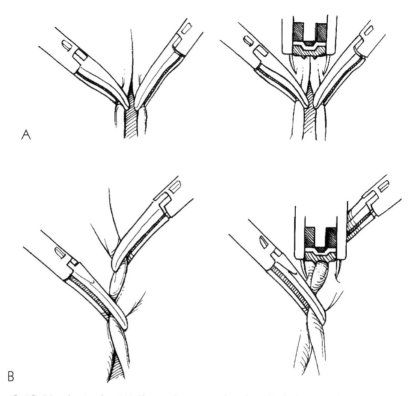

Fig. 3-12. Hernia stapler. **(A)** Tip-to-tip approximation: Both tissue edges are approximated by placing the graspers tip to tip. **(B)** The X arrangement: The tissue flaps cross over for a distance of 1 to 1.5 cm. The tissue edges are approximated at the point where the edges cross. (*Figure continues.*)

lengths. The 30-mm version is suitable for dividing a vascular pedicle or the small bowel. The 60-mm version is for dividing colon or stomach, or for making a side-to-side anastomosis (e.g., gastrojejunostomy). In some situations, the 60-mm linear cutter is too big to handle comfortably, so two or more fires of the 30-mm device can be used in sequence.

The degree of compression of opposing structures is determined by the staple depth. Shallower staples (1 mm) give a tighter compression and are used for blood vessels, while looser compression (1.5 and 2 mm) is used for the gut. The cartridges are color coded: white for vascular work, blue for the intestine, and green for something thicker, such as the stomach. A gauge is available to measure tissue thickness to select the appropriate cartridge, although most laparoscopic surgeons do not routinely use it.

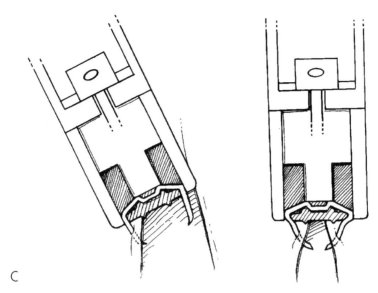

C

Fig. 3-12. (*Continued*). **(C)** The handles of the stapler are squeezed enough to deploy the staple partially from the jaws. One tip is pushed into the tissue, the opposite edge is pulled into position, and the staple is completely fired.

Port Sites for Linear Cutters   A 12-mm cannula is needed for the 30-mm linear cutter, while a 15- or 18-mm cannula is needed for the 60-mm version. The cannula must be far enough from the surgical site to allow the jaws of the linear cutter to get entirely within the abdomen and free enough from the cannula so they can open. The angle of approach to the operating site should also be considered, especially when applying a linear cutter to a relatively immobile tissue, such as the splenic hilar vessels. The device should approach perpendicular to the structure to be divided, and the jaws of the instrument should be in full view as they close.

Proper Use of the Linear Cutter   The structure to be divided should be mobilized circumferentially. Note that the staple line is shorter than the cartridge, and the cut is shorter than the staple line, so the tissue bundle must be shorter than the cartridge (and shorter than the length of the cut).

The jaws must be passed around the tissue and closed; clearance along both sides must be checked, and then the jaws are fired (Fig. 3-13A). Some 60-mm linear cutters are equipped with power firing, which uses compressed air to deliver the staples and the blade. The jaws are opened, and the tissue is released. Then the jaws are closed again (so they will pass through the port), and the instrument is withdrawn from the abdomen. The integrity of the staple line on both sides is confirmed. Minor oozing of blood usually stops within a few minutes.[41] The linear cutter can then be reloaded with another cartridge if needed.

The technique for a bowel anastomosis[42] (e.g., gastrojejunostomy) is as follows. The proximal jejunum is aligned against the greater curvature of the antrum, and stay sutures are placed at either extreme of the planned anastomosis. Small enterotomies are placed at one end, and the jaws of the 60-mm linear cutter are placed into the stomach and jejunum. Access is easier from the left, but space is tight. After making sure that mesentery and omentum will not be included, the device is closed and fired. The jaws are opened, and any bleeding points are cauterized along the staple line (i.e., inside the lumen). The enterotomies are closed by deploying the stapler again or by suturing (Fig. 3-13B). If there is not enough room to use the 60-mm stapler, the 30-mm stapler should be used twice to get an equivalent result.

Circular Staplers

Circular staplers available in diameters ranging from 21 to 31 mm are used for low colonic anastomoses. In a laparoscopic-assisted colectomy, once the colon is divided distal to the lesion with a linear cutter, the proximal stump is pulled through a trocar site that has been enlarged. The resection is completed outside the abdominal cavity, and the anvil of the stapler is inserted into the proximal stump and is secured with a purse-string suture. This is returned to the abdomen, and the pneumoperitoneum is reestablished. Then the stapler, with its shaft retracted, is passed up the rectum. When the head of the instrument reaches the top of the rectal stump, the shaft is advanced by turning the knob. The tip is positioned next to the staple line, and then the wall is pierced; the shaft is further advanced by unwinding the knob until the marker on the shaft is visible outside the bowel. The tip should be detached, which reveals a hollow shaft. A suture passed through the tip will facilitate its removal through a cannula. The shaft and the anvil are joined (Fig. 3-14), and the knob is turned to retract the shaft until a marker indicates they are close enough. Details of this scenario depend on minor differences in the instruments as described in Chapter 2. The surgeon checks to make sure no other tissue is caught in the device and fires it. The knob is unwound to release the jaws, and the stapler is withdrawn with a gentle back and forth twisting motion.

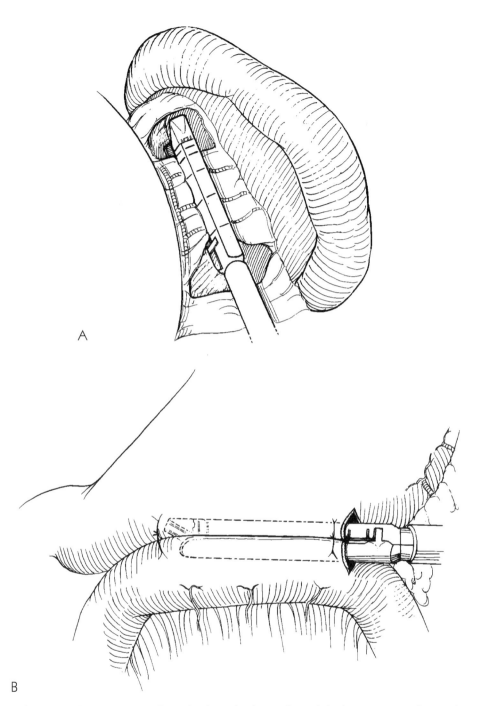

Fig. 3-13. Linear cutter. **(A)** Once the tissue has been cleared, the jaws are passed around the tissue and closed, clearance along both sides is checked, and the cutter is fired. **(B)** A linear cutter is also used for bowel anastomosis. When the jaws are introduced, they should not be moved back and forth, because this movement may tear the wall.

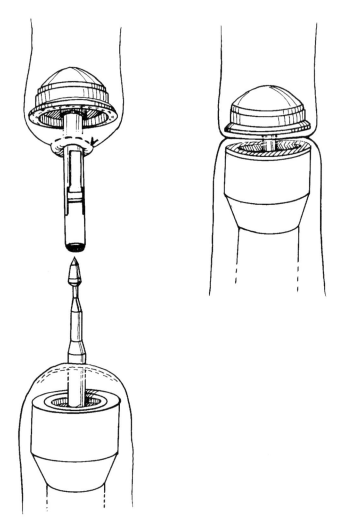

Fig. 3-14. Circular stapler. When the shaft of the handle and the anvil are joined, the anvil and trocar should be lined up correctly.

The surgeon should make sure that there are two complete tissue rings in the device and inspects the anastomosis for bleeding or gaps. Additional sutures may be placed, if necessary. The integrity of the anastomosis may be tested by placing a noncrushing clamp proximal to the anastomosis and instilling air or water into the rectum.

Although technically more demanding, the procedure can also be performed entirely intracorporeally. The specimen is removed through the rectum, and the circular stapling device with its anvil is passed through the rectum into the abdominal cavity. The anvil is dislodged and secured by a purse-string suture into the proximal stump.

Irrigators and Aspirators

Irrigation and aspiration devices help to keep the operating site clear. Unlike open surgery, small amounts of blood may obscure the operating field, and wiping with a gauze sponge is unwieldy.

When setting up the device, the surgeon should make sure that it is connected to the vacuum and that the irrigant bag and switches work. The irrigation fluid most commonly used is normal saline or lactated Ringer's solution with 5000 U/L heparin (to prevent clot formation, because clots are difficult to aspirate). The surgeon should avoid getting the scope too close to the operating field when irrigating, because the lens may get splashed. When a close view is needed (e.g., when identifying a bleeding spot), the laparoscope can be moved closer after the bleeding spot is flooded with irrigant. The puddle is aspirated slowly, and the bleeder can be seen. The pneumoperitoneum will be lost quickly—along with the exposure—if the aspirator is out of the fluid, and even high-flow insufflators cannot keep up. This may be deliberate and helpful if the intention is to evacuate accumulated smoke, but most often it is accidental and a nuisance.

Activating the suction close to fatty tissue or other mobile structures may lead to clogging of the channel. If this happens, the irrigation switch should be pressed briefly, and the channel will clear.

At the end of the operation, blood and irrigation fluid should be removed. If the dissection has been extensive (e.g., colectomy), the area may be irrigated thoroughly to remove small pieces of fat or clots. The dependent part of the abdomen should also be checked when the patient has been tilted during the procedure.

Electrocautery

Monopolar Electrocautery

The principles of electrosurgery, and in particular the risks associated with laparoscopy, should be reviewed (Ch. 2) before using a monopolar electrosurgical device. Cautery is used for cutting and coagulating. The four most commonly used electrode configurations are hook, spatula, point, and ball, and laparoscopic instruments such as scissors, dissectors, and graspers may also be connected to an electrosurgical generator.

Before use, the insulation of the electrosurgical instrument is checked by inspecting the surface for defects. Cautery instruments should not be used with a metal cannula that has been isolated from the abdominal wall with a plastic sleeve, because a charge will be induced in the cannula. Also the instrument must not be activated until it touches the tissue. The whole of the uninsulated tip of the electrode should always be visible during use. Care should be taken when using the electrode near metal clips or other metal instruments, because of the risk of direct coupling whereby the clip or instrument becomes electrically hot. This is one cause of biliary stricture formation (see Ch. 9).

Use of the Hook, Spatula, Point, and Ball Electrodes The point and hook electrodes should be used like a scalpel, adhering to the principles of optimal exposure. The tissue should be under traction and countertraction immediately around the area to be dissected to reduce the likelihood of cutting adjacent or underlying structures. The electrode should be activated only on contact with the tissue. A cutting waveform is used to incise relatively avascular tissue, such as peritoneum, while a coagulating waveform is often more suited to incising vascular tissue, such as liver. The dissection is begun on a low-power setting (30 to 40 watts), and the power is gradually increased to achieve the desired tissue effect. The hook electrode is specially suited to cutting a layer of tissue while avoiding injury to underlying structures (Fig. 3-15A). This is done by separating the tissue to be cut from whatever is beneath it by blunt dissection. The tissue is captured in the concavity of the hook electrode, and the current is delivered to transect the tissue.

The spatula electrode may be used as a coagulator, a scalpel, or a blunt dissector. It is good for dissecting the gallbladder from the liver bed (Fig. 3-15B).

The ball electrode is used, as in open surgery, to coagulate a diffusely bleeding area of tissue (e.g., liver bed), but it should be used sparingly and cautiously. Tamponade of the tissue with forceps or gauze is often preferred.

Electrosurgical current may be transmitted through conventional instruments such as graspers, dissectors, and scissors. A bleeding vessel may be grasped and coagulated. Electrocautery is a valuable enhancement for scissors because it adds a coagulating function to the mechanical cutting action of the scissors. Because most scissors have a fairly long uninsulated segment, the

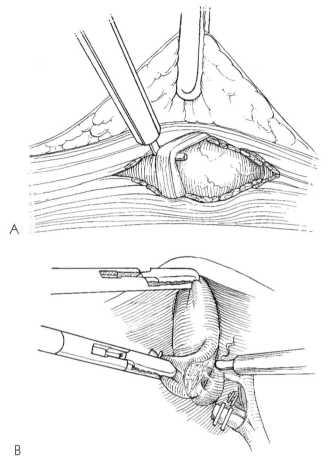

Fig. 3-15. Electrocautery. (**A**) The hook cautery is activated after the tissue is dissected into its concavity. (**B**) The spatula can also be used as a blunt dissector, thus optimizing the exposure for the next segment of dissection.

most proximal extent of which may be off screen, the surgeon must be especially careful to avoid accidental coagulation of tissues.

Bipolar Electrocautery

When using a bipolar instrument, the current is transmitted only through the tissue between the jaws of the instrument. Hence the tissue may be coagulated safely with less risk of injury to underlying or adjacent tissue. For bipolar instruments, a generator specifically adapted to the delivery of bipolar current is used.

The most commonly used bipolar instrument is Kleppinger forceps, which is used to control bleeding in a similar fashion to that described for monopolar instruments.

Bipolar scissors may be used to combine a mechanical cutting action with a hemostatic effect. This is an especially useful way of incising tissue, such as gallbladder peritoneum or the seromuscular layer of gut, where underlying gallbladder or gut mucosa must not be perforated. The tissue to be incised is placed between the jaws of the scissors and the current activated. Once the tissue is seen to whiten, the handles of the scissors are compressed to close the jaws and mechanically cut the tissue. The hemostasis takes a few seconds longer than when using a monopolar instrument in similar fashion.

Self-Retaining Arm

A self-retaining arm (mechanical assistant) may be useful to hold the laparoscope or retractors if repositioning is infrequent. These devices should be placed so they do not limit the movement of other instruments.

When using a self-retaining arm to hold a liver retractor during gastroesophageal procedures, the base is clamped to the rail on the side of the operating table at *midchest level* so the arm can course along the right flank to reach the retractor without encroaching on the operating field. Placing the base too low on the table forces the arm to arch up into the field before it gets to the retractor. When using a self-retaining arm to hold the scope, the device should have an arch large enough to allow free movement of operating instruments.

If correctly used, self-retaining arms can provide consistent, less traumatic retraction of the organ and a stable view of the surgical field.

Technical Notes

Any laparoscopic procedure depends critically on exposure. If exposure is adequate, the operation is greatly simplified. In this section, the techniques of dissection are discussed.

Handling and Dissection of Soft Tissue

For exposure, soft tissues, such as intestine, can be safely grasped by an atraumatic grasper, such as a Babcock or Glassmann clamp, if a generous amount of the tissue is grasped and force is minimal. Traction should be perpendicular to the dissection plane. The operating port should be selected so that the operating instrument approaches the operative site at a 30° to 60° angle relative to the scope. If the soft tissue is pulled in the wrong direction, the field will be eclipsed. This can also result from inserting the instrument through the wrong port.

The peritoneum is usually incised sharply, either with scissors or electrocautery. Techniques of blunt dissection of a loose connective tissue plane between organs are as follows. First, a dissector is pushed against the tissue with its jaws closed, and the tissues are dissected by opening the jaws (Fig. 3-16A). Alternatively, a small amount of the tissue is grasped and pulled (Fig. 3-16B). This technique is also useful to strip a blood vessel or tubular structure, such as the cystic duct. For areolar connective tissue, such as in the mediastinum or preperitoneal space, the tip of the instrument is raked through the tissue after the position of the plane is estimated from visual inspection (Fig. 3-16C).

Scissors or electrocautery may also be used (but not blindly) for small (e.g., 1-mm) pieces of tissue that can be clearly seen to be dispensable. Scissors have the advantage that they can also be used for blunt dissection or cautery, and their wider versatility has led to their being favored by many experienced laparoscopic surgeons. Early in the surgeon's experience, other instruments are easier to use and probably safer.

Blood Vessels

Dissection of Blood Vessels

Blood vessels are often buried in connective tissue. The first step is to identify the vessel from the surrounding tissue, which is most easily done by placing traction in a direction that stretches the vessel longitudinally. The blood vessel can also be grasped by an atraumatic grasper and pulled to the proper tension.

A port should be used that allows the dissecting instrument to approach the vessel perpendicularly. Blunt dissection should be performed along the surface of the vessel (Fig. 3-17A). The jaws of scissors and tip of the hook or spatula cautery can also be used for blunt dissection. Cautery should be activated only when the tip of the electrode is visible and the tissue inside the hook is not a blood vessel larger than 1 mm in diameter.

Laparoscopic ultrasonography may prove to be a help in detecting blood vessels buried in connective tissue. The ultrasonic dissector (CUSA) has been

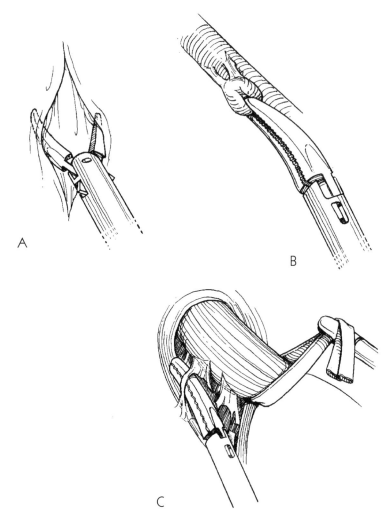

Fig. 3-16. Dissection of soft tissue by a dissector. (**A**) A dissector is pushed against the tissue with its jaws closed. The tissue is dissected by opening the jaws. (**B**) Plucking: A small amount of the tissue is grasped and pulled by a dissector. (**C**) Raking: The tip of the instrument is raked through the tissue after the direction of the plane is estimated visually.

shown to be able to dissect blood vessels from surrounding fatty tissues without injuring them (see Ch. 2).

A circumferential window must be developed around the vessel, and if the vessel is bigger than 1 to 2 mm the surface can be stripped clean of connective

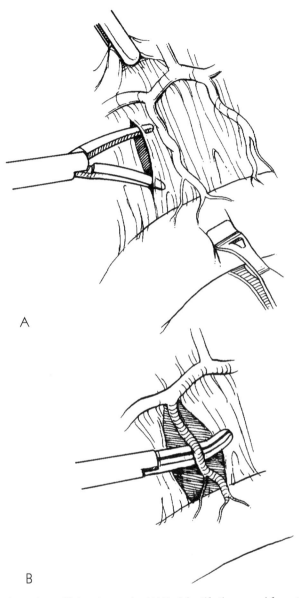

A

B

Fig. 3-17. Dissection of blood vessels. **(A)** To identify the vessel from the surrounding tissue, traction is placed in a direction that stretches it longitudinally. The port is selected so that the operating instrument approaches the vessel perpendicularly. Blunt dissection is then performed along the surface of the vessels. **(B)** For vessels larger than 1 to 2 mm, a circumferential window should be developed around the vessel, stripping it until the adventitia is clean. A forceps can then be passed behind the vessel so the tips appear on the other side.

tissue. Smaller vessels (e.g., short gastrics) should be allowed to retain a thin layer of connective tissue or else they may be torn during the dissection. When the dissection is adequate, a forceps can be passed behind the vessel so the tips appear on the other side (Fig. 3-17B). The window can then be enlarged along the axis of the vessel by moving the forceps or hook cautery back and forth. When enough length is clean, clips are applied and the vessel divided.

Preventing and Controlling Bleeding

In open surgery, small amounts of bleeding are no problem. Blood and clots can be wiped away easily, and hemostasis can be obtained by just applying compression manually. Suction can be unrestrained, because there is no pneumoperitoneum to worry about, and the bleeding site can be pinpointed quickly. In contrast, in laparoscopic surgery, even small amounts of bleeding are a real nuisance, because the blood obscures its source, illumination decreases as the blood absorbs light, and the use of suction must be rationed so exposure is not lost. Finally, any blood splashed on the end of the scope blanks out the image. As with any difficulty in laparoscopic surgery, exposure is critical for controlling bleeding.

If bleeding occurs, the surgeon should never apply clips or cautery blindly. Small amounts of bleeding usually stop spontaneously or following pressure applied for 30 to 60 seconds with forceps or a small roll of gauze. The area should then be cleared by irrigation and suction, and the point of bleeding identified. A small rolled-up gauze sponge is useful to clear blood clots. If bleeding persists, it is most easily stopped by cauterizing the exact spot or applying a clip. Sometimes the best strategy is to grasp the site with forceps and touch the cautery to the forceps. When applying clips, the "half-way squeezed clip" (teardrop) technique can be useful (see the section *Clip Appliers*, above). More serious bleeding that cannot be managed by these techniques is discussed in Chapter 6 and may require that the abdomen be opened.

Removal of Specimen

On completion of a laparoscopic resection, retrieval of the tissue is a step for which techniques and devices have been specifically developed. The two important issues are whether the tissue is small enough to be retrieved through a port or, in the case of malignancy or infected tissue, the risk of seeding tumor cells or microorganisms at the trocar site.[43–45] If the specimen is small enough and is not infected or malignant, it may be removed through a cannula. Any infected or malignant tissue should be enclosed in a retrieval bag before removal. Retrieval bags are commercially available. The polyurethane bags are porous to particles smaller than 0.5 μm, and so it is theoretically better to use an impervious nylon bag for removing infected or malignant tissue.

Techniques for Tissue Removal

If the specimen is not infected or malignant, and it is too large for the cannula, the simplest method is to remove it through a port site that has been surgically enlarged. One retrieval technique is to grasp the tissue (e.g., gallbladder) with a grasper inserted through the midline cannula. Keeping a firm grasp on the tissue, the grasper, cannula, and tissue are pulled through the skin incision using a gentle twisting action. This may bring just a small part of specimen through the skin. In this case, it should be secured with Alice clamps and the lumen opened. Aspirating bile and removing gallstones may be enough to permit an unrestricted extraction. If gallstones are too large to be retrieved through this opening, they may be crushed using forceps inserted into the gallbladder through this opening. If stones are too hard to be crushed and still too big to fit through the wound, the fascial defect should be enlarged bluntly or with scissors. A small specimen enclosed in a bag (e.g., the appendix) can be retrieved in similar fashion. In this case, the bag should be partly removed and then opened to decompress trapped carbon dioxide from within the bag.[46]

For a specimen larger than 2 to 3 cm in diameter (e.g., spleen, kidney, colon, or ovarian mass), the alternatives are to perform a minilaparotomy, to remove the tissue through the cul de sac of the vagina or the rectum (for anterior resections), or to remove it piecemeal.

Laparotomy is conveniently performed through one of the cannula sites, either using a muscle-splitting gridiron incision, a vertical incision through the linea alba, or a Pfannenstiel incision. In laparoscopic colon resections accompanied by a colostomy, the specimen may be removed through the colostomy site. The advantage of performing a laparotomy is that it is easy, and the specimen can be removed intact. The disadvantage is that it may theoretically negate some of the benefits of the minimally invasive surgery. In a laparoscopic colectomy, the specimen can be removed transrectally. In laparoscopic gynecologic procedures, the specimen may be retrieved through the incision made transvaginally in the anterior fornix.

Devices for Tissue Retrieval

The simplest retrieval devices are a finger of a surgeon's glove, a sterile condom, or sterile plastic bag. A polyurethane bag is available that has a ring around the entrance, which holds the mouth of the bag open, so it is easier to insert a specimen (see Fig. 2-14). Once the specimen is in the bag, the ring is detached, and the mouth is closed by cinching up a drawstring. The bag and its contents are then pulled through the opening in the abdominal wall. These bags reduce the likelihood of spillage. The bags are small (6 × 2.5 inches) and made of polyurethane and thus only suitable for removing small specimens (e.g., appendix or gallbladder). For larger specimens that require debulking, a nylon bag that is resistant to tearing should be used.

It may be technically demanding to get the organ into the bag. The spleen, for example, is a real challenge. The hilar structures or a piece of the soft tissue resected with the specimen should be grabbed and used as a handle. Another trick is to tie an umbilical tape snugly around the spleen and use the tape as a handle. The spleen is then put into the bag, taking care to avoid breaking the capsule, which may result in splenosis (Fig. 3-18).

If the organ requires debulking, the mouth of the bag is exteriorized through one of the port sites that has been enlarged, and a forceps (e.g., sponge forceps) is introduced through the mouth to extract the organ piecemeal. Alternatively, a commercially available morcellator may be used to debulk the tissue. The drawback of this maneuver is that the specimen is much harder for the pathologist to analyze.

Tissue Approximation

Tissue approximation remains one of the most difficult technical challenges in laparoscopic surgery. Although the technique is not identical to that in open surgery, the principles should be the same. Techniques and instruments for laparoscopic suturing are available (see Ch. 4), but laparoscopic suturing is technically more demanding than can be practically used for hand-sewn anastomosis of the gut. Stapling devices have been modified for laparoscopic use

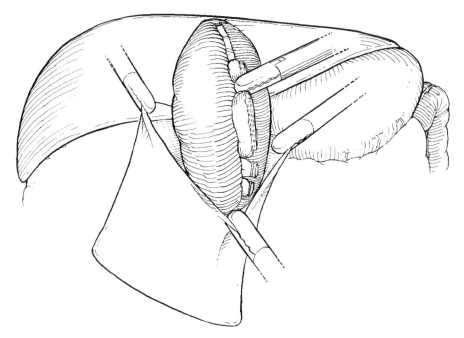

Fig. 3-18. Tissue retrieval. When retrieving the spleen, the hilar structures or a piece of soft tissue resected with the specimen should be grabbed and used as a handle.

and used for a variety of operations. It is still mandatory for laparoscopic surgeons to be able to place stitches and tie knots. Bowel anastomoses, for example, may be performed using linear cutters, and the residual enterotomy can also be closed with a stapling device. Nevertheless, it is often necessary to place additional interrupted sutures to close any gaps left during the mechanically performed anastomosis.[47]

Mechanical approximation of tissues has not always been used appropriately and may have occasionally lead to complications. Hernia staplers, for example, have been used inappropriately as an alternative to suturing for reapproximating the gut. Shortcuts like this are inexcusable.

In general, tissue approximation and anastomoses in laparoscopic surgery should be performed similar to open surgery and their principles should not be compromised. A new procedure should not be performed until it is shown to be safe and effective in animals. The surgeon must be particularly aware of the risk of tissue ischemia if stapling devices are used inappropriately, if leakage occurs, or if suturing is performed inadequately.

Exiting the Abdomen

Inspection of the Abdominal Cavity

On completing a laparoscopic procedure, the abdominal cavity is inspected for bleeding or visceral injury. If bleeding is a concern, the intra-abdominal pressure should be decreased to about 5 mmHg,[48] which eliminates the venous tamponading effect of the standard 15 mmHg pneumoperitoneum.

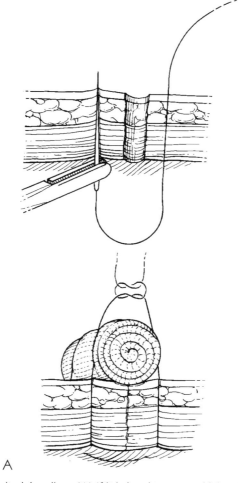

A

Fig. 3-19. Cannula site bleeding. (**A**) If it is hard to control bleeding, a through-and-through stitch may be placed. The suture may be tied over a piece of gauze. (*Figure continues.*)

Removal of Cannulas and Evacuation of the Peritoneal Cavity

Once everything is shipshape, the cannulas can be removed. All cannulas except the one for the laparoscope should be removed under direct observation. If there is a 5-mm port, a 5-mm laparoscope may be inserted through it so that the 10-mm ports, which are more likely to be the site of bleeding, can be inspected.[49]

As the cannula is pulled out, the hole should be plugged with a finger so the pneumoperitoneum is maintained. The cannula site is inspected from the inside, and if bleeding is observed, hemostasis can be obtained with the electrocautery or by placing a stitch. If it is hard to control bleeding, a through-and-through stitch may be placed. The suture may be tied outside over a gauze bolster or sponge pledget (Fig. 3-19A).[50] If done correctly, bleeding should rarely persist. Another method, which can be used for bleeding during an operation, is to insert a Foley catheter through the port site wound, inflate the balloon within the abdomen, and place it on traction, so the balloon tamponades the bleeding vessel. The balloon catheter is anchored in place with a Kelly clamp at the skin level (Fig. 3-19B). Although it usually is needed only temporarily (i.e., during the operation), this catheter may be left in place overnight.[51,52]

The last cannula through which the laparoscope has been placed is withdrawn with the laparoscope inside the cannula so the tract can be observed. If there is bleeding from this wound that cannot be controlled with electro-

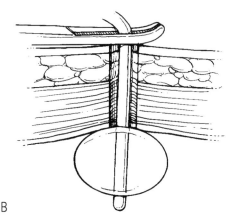

B

Fig. 3-19 (*Continued*). **(B)** For cannula site bleeding, a large Foley catheter is inserted through the port site wound, the balloon is inflated within the abdomen, and the catheter is placed on traction.

cautery or stitches, cannulas can be reintroduced through the other port sites, and a through-and-through suture can be placed. This is a rare problem.

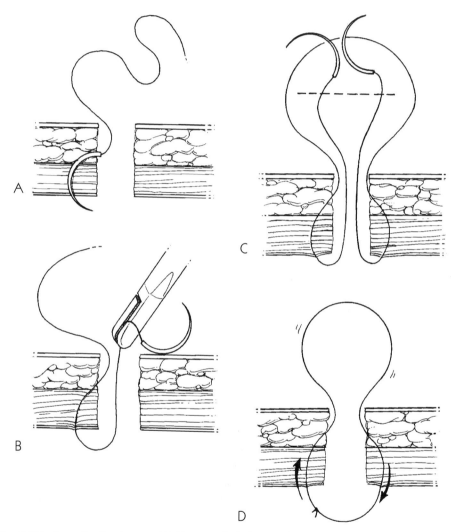

Fig. 3-20. Cannula site closure. (**A**) The needle is inserted into the abdomen including the abdominal wall. (**B**) Once the needle is inside the abdominal cavity, a laparoscopic forceps is passed into the abdomen, through the cannula wound, and the thread is grabbed next to the needle to pull it out. (**C**) The other needle is then driven into the other edge of the wound and pulled out like the first one. Both needles are removed, the ends of suture are tied, and the knot is dropped in the abdomen to create a loop including both edges of the wound with the knot within the abdominal cavity. (**D**) The suture is rotated to pull the knot out through one side of the wound. (*Figure continues.*)

As the last cannula is removed, the pneumoperitoneum is totally evacuated. If a pneumoscrotum is present, it should be manually decompressed. The surgeon should confirm that no bowel or omentum is trapped in the cannula site wound after removing the last cannula.

Cannula Site Closure

Cannula sites larger than 5 mm should be closed to prevent hernia formation, especially in the lower abdomen.[53,54] Many ways of closing the cannula site wound have been described either with or without maintaining the pneumoperitoneum. For maximum effectiveness, the suture must be full thickness and include the fascia, muscle, and peritoneum. It is difficult to impossible, however, to place a suture through the small port site skin incision that includes the full thickness of the musculofascial abdominal wall. Thus, the larger cannula sites, especially below the umbilicus, should be closed under direct vision with the aid of the laparoscope.[48]

An 0-Maxon or PDS on a straight or curved needle is most commonly used. It is usually easy to drive a needle from outside into the abdominal cavity, but it is not always as easy to drive the needle from the inside and make it come out where you want. For placing a full-thickness stitch, it may be helpful to place Sinn retractors on the skin and subcutaneous fat tissue to expose the fascia or to lift up the apex of the incision with two single-prong skin hooks. There are several easy ways to place a full-thickness stitch.

In one technique, a needle is driven into the abdomen, grabbed by an instrument introduced through the wound being closed, and pulled outside (Fig. 3-20A & B). The needle is threaded on the other end of the suture and is then driven through the other edge of the wound into the abdomen, and it is pulled out like the first one. Both needles are then removed, and the ends of the suture are tied. The knot is dropped in the abdomen, so there is now a loop including both edges of the wound with the knot within the abdominal cavity (Fig. 3-20C). The loop is

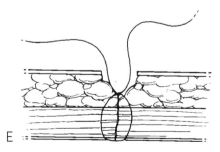

Fig. 3-20 (Continued). **(E)** The knot is cut out and the suture is tied to close the wound securely.

then rotated to pull the knot out through one side of the wound (Fig. 3-20D). The knot is cut out and the suture retied to close the wound securely with the knot on the outside (Fig. 3-20E).

A Keith needle or other needle with large turning radius can also be used to traverse the fascia and the peritoneum. It, however, requires an additional port to introduce a laparoscopic needle driver to drive the needle from the inside. If it is difficult to make the needle come out in the correct position, a large hollow needle (e.g., 14 G) should be inserted outside-in to direct the exit of the Keith needle from the abdominal cavity. Both needles are then pulled out together.

There are also specially designed devices that can be used to place these sutures.[55] They work well, but they also add another little expense to the case. One version resembles a crochet hook inside a needle; another one is a needle-nosed forceps that grips the suture. The device is loaded with a suture and inserted into the abdomen adjacent to the wound. The suture is detached from the device in the abdominal cavity, and the device is withdrawn. Then it is inserted through the opposite side of the wound and used to grasp and pull the suture through.

Placing sutures in the absence of a pneumoperitoneum is not unlike wound closure in open surgery. It is often impossible, however, to place a precise full-thickness stitch without the pneumoperitoneum, so this method is only suited for closing of upper abdominal port site wounds not larger than 10 mm.

Summary

Performing laparoscopic surgery safely depends on the appropriate use of instruments that have been specially designed for these tasks. In addition, new principles must be learned (especially trocar placement) and new skills developed (especially suturing and two-handed surgery). This chapter identifies some of the important operative techniques with which a surgeon must be familiar before undertaking a laparoscopic procedure.

References

1. Semm K: Endoscopic Intraabdominal Surgery. Christian-Albrects-Universität, Kiel, Germany, 1984
2. Cuschieri A, Berci G: Laparoscopic Biliary Surgery. p. 15. Blackwell Scientific, London, 1990

3. Lee VS, Chari RS, Cucchiaro G et al: Complications of laparoscopic cholecystectomy. Am J Surg 165:527, 1993

4. Katkhouda N, Mouiel J: A new technique of surgical treatment of chronic duodenal ulcer without laparotomy by videocoelioscopy. Am J Surg 161:361, 1991

5. Bagnato VJ: Laparoscopic Nissen fundoplication. Surg Laparosc Endosc 2:188, 1992

6. Soper NJ: Laparoscopic cholecystectomy. Curr Probl Surg 28:581, 1991

7. Nogueras JJ, Wexner SD: Laparoscopic colon resection. Perspect Colon Rectal Surg 5:79, 1992

8. Geis WP, Coletta AV, Verdeja JC et al: Sequential psychomotor skills development in laparoscopic colon surgery. Arch Surg 129:206, 1994

9. Sackier JM: Laparoscopy: applications to colorectal surgery. Semin Colon Rectal Surg 3:2, 1992

10. Hinder RA, Filipi CJ: The technique of laparoscopic Nissen fundoplication. Surg Laparosc Endosc 2:265, 1992

11. Kuster GG, Gilroy S: Laparoscopic technique for repair of paraesophageal hiatal hernias. J Laparoendosc Surg 3:331, 1993

12. Nowzaradan Y, Barnes JP, Jr, Westmoreland J et al: Laparoscopic appendectomy: treatment of choice for suspected appendicitis. Surg Laparosc Endosc 3:411, 1993

13. Gajraj H, el-Din A, McGuiness C et al: Technique for laparoscopic appendicectomy, letter; comment. Br J Surg 79:1246, 1992

14. Fowler DL, White SA: Laparoscopy-assisted sigmoid resection. Surg Laparosc Endosc 1:183, 1991

15. Phillips EH, Franklin M, Carrol BJ: Laparoscopic colectomy. Ann Surg 216:703, 1992

16. Dallamgne B, Weerts JM, Jehaes C et al: Laparoscopic Nissen fundoplication: preliminary report. Surg Laparosc Endosc 3:138, 1991

17. Cuschieri A: Laparoscopic ligamentum teres (round ligament) cardiopexy. p. 378. In Berci G (ed): Problems in General Surgery. JB Lippincott, Philadelphia

18. Jacobs M, Verdeja JC, Goldstein DS: Minimally invasive colon resection (laparoscopic colectomy). Surg Laparosc Endosc 1:144, 1991

19. Cuschieri A, Shimi S, Nathanson LK: Laparoscopic reduction, crural repair, and fundoplication of large hiatal hernia. Am J Surg 163:425, 1992

20. Sackier JM: Laparoscopic colon and rectal surgery. p. 179. In Hunter JG, Sackier JM (eds): Minimally Invasive Surgery. McGraw-Hill, New York.

21. McKernan JB: Laparoscopic cholecystectomy. Am Surg 57(5):309, 1991

22. White JV: Registry of laparoscopic cholecystectomy and new and evolving laparoscopic techniques. Am J Surg 165:536, 1993

23. Gotz F, Pier A, Bacher C: Modified laparoscopic appendectomy in surgery. Surg Endosc 4:6, 1990

24. Daniel JF, Gurley LD, Kurtz BR et al: The use of an automatic stapling device for laparoscopic appendectomy. Obstet Gynecol 78:721, 1991

25. Zucker KA, Bailey RW, Gadacz TR et al: Laparoscopic guided cholecystectomy. Am J Surg 161:36, 1991

26. Reddick EJ: An Introductory Course in Laparoscopic Surgery. 2nd Ed. EJR Enterprises, Chicago, 1990

27. Hoffman HC, Traverso AL: Preperitoneal herniorrhaphy. One surgeon's successful technique. Arch Surg 128:969, 1993

28. McKernan JB, Laws HL: Laparoscopic Nissen fundoplication for the treatment of gastroesophageal reflux disease. Am Surg 60:87, 1994

29. Kavoussi LR, Soper NJ: Establishing the pneumoperitoneum. p. 34. In Soper NJ, Odem RR, Clayman RV et al (eds): Essential of Laparoscopy. Quality Medical Publishing, St. Louis, MO, 1994

30. Colver RM: Laparoscopy: basic technique, instrumentation, and complications. Surg Laparosc Endosc 2:35, 1992

31. Bailey RW: Complications of laparoscopic general surgery. p. 318. In Zucker K (ed): Surgical Laparoscopy. Quality Medical Publishing, St. Louis, MO, 1991

32. Winfield HN: Abdominal access: initial trocar placement. p. 48. In Soper NJ, Odem RR, Clayman RV et al (eds): Essential of Laparoscopy. Quality Medical Publishing, St. Louis, MO, 1994

33. Hasson HM: Open laparoscopy vs. closed laparoscopy: a comparison of complication rates. Adv Planned Parenthood 13:41, 1978

34. Riedel HH, Willenbrock-Lehnmann E, Mecke H et al: The frequency of distribution of various pelvioscopic (laparoscopic) operations, including complication rates. Statistics of the Federal Republic of Germany in the years 1983–1985. Zentralbl Gynakol 111:78, 1989

35. Kaali SG, Vartfai G: Direct insertion of the laparoscopic trocar after an earlier laparotomy. J Reprod Med 33:739, 1988

36. Fitzgibbons RJ, Jr, Salerno GM, Filipi CJ: Open laparoscopy. p. 87. In Zucker K (ed): Surgical Laparoscopy. Quality Medical Publishing, St. Louis, MO, 1991

37. Copeland C, Wing R, Hulka JF: Direct trocar insertion at laparoscopy: an evaluation. Obstet Gynecol 62:655, 1983

38. Brown AS, Mueller PR, Ferruci JT, Jr: Controlled percutaneous gastrostomy: nylon T-fastener for fixation of the anterior gastric wall. Radiology 158:543, 1986

39. Duh QY, Way LW: Laparoscopic gastrostomy using T-fasteners as retractors and anchors. Surg Endosc 7:60, 1993

40. Duh QY, Way LW: Laparoscopic jejunostomy using T-fasteners as retractors and anchors. Arch Surg 128:105, 1993

41. Lefor AT, Melvin WS, Bailey RW, et al: Laparoscopic splenectomy in management of immune thrombocytopenia purpura. Surgery 114:613, 1994

42. Lointier P, Leroux S, Ferrier C et al: A technique of laparoscopic gastrectomy and Billroth II gastrojejunostomy. J Laparosc Surg 3:353, 1993

43. Scoggin SD, Frazee RC, Snyder SK et al: Laparoscopic assisted bowel surgery. Dis Colon Rectum 36:747, 1993

44. Alexander RJ, Jacques BC, Mitchell KG: Laparoscopically assisted colectomy and wound recurrence. Lancet 341:249, 1993

45. Diettrich NA, Kaplan G: Laparoscopic surgery for HIV-infected patients: minimizing dangers for all concerned. J Laparoendosc Surg 1(5):295, 1991

46. O'Reilly MJ, Reddick EJ, Miller WD, Saye WB. Laparoscopic appendectomy. p. 301. In Zucker KA (ed): Surgical Laparoscopy Update. Quality Medical Publishing, St. Louis, MO, 1993

47. Brune IB, Scholenben K: Laparoscopic side to side gastrojejunostomy. Chirurg 63:577, 1992

48. Winfield HN, Clayman RV: Exiting the abdomen. p. 204. In Soper NJ, Odem RR, Clayman RV et al (eds): Essential of Laparoscopy. Quality Medical Publishing, St. Louis, MO, 1994

49. Plaus WJ: Laparoscopic trocar site hernias. J Laparoendosc Surg 3:567, 1993

50. Kent RB, 3d, Kent RB, Jr: Control of hemorrhage from a trocar site. Surg Laparosc Endosc 3:225, 1993

51. Boswell WC, Odom JW, Rudolph R et al: A method for controlling bleeding from abdominal wall puncture after laparoscopic surgery. Surg Laparosc Endosc 3:47, 1993

52. Burney TL, Campbell EC, Jr, Naslund MJ et al: Complications of staging laparoscopic pelvic lymphadenectomy. Surg Laparosc Endosc 3:184, 1993

53. Schlossnickel B, Leibl B, Bittner R: Incarcerated scar hernia in an adjacent channel after laparoscopic cholecystectomy—a rare complication? Chirurg 64:666, 1993

54. Hass BE, Schrager RE: Small bowel obstruction due to Richter's hernia after laparoscopic procedures. J Laparoendosc Surg 3:421, 1993

55. Phillips JM: Laparoscopy. Williams & Wilkins, Baltimore, 1977

Suturing

Z. Szabo

SUTURING, ONE OF MANKIND'S EARLIEST CRAFTS, HAS UNDERGONE periodic changes over the years to meet new challenges. In open surgery, suturing techniques reached their modern form after the turn of the century, when Carel and Guthrie developed precision methods for use in vascular surgery.[1] In minimal access surgery, suturing and knotting was attempted by the early pioneers,[2,3] but the techniques have improved substantially since.

Initially, knotting was mainly accomplished extracorporeally by bringing the ends of the threads out through the cannula, tying a knot, and then pushing it back in and down onto the tissues. This technique is most practical for large sturdy tissues, however, and it is time-consuming. For small delicate tissues, extracorporeal knotting is clumsy and less satisfactory. In this situation, intracorporeal knotting using fine, needle holders, sutures, and suturing style are necessary.[4,5] Anyone involved in advanced laparoscopic surgery should be able to suture and tie knots entirely intracorporeally.

Three considerations are particularly important when learning how to suture: the set-up, visual perception, and eye-hand coordination.

Set-Up

The surgeon's position in relation to the instruments and prospective suture line is very influential in determining the result. The two most critical concerns are (1) coaxial alignment of the visual path and (2) triangulation of the camera and operating ports (Fig. 4-1).

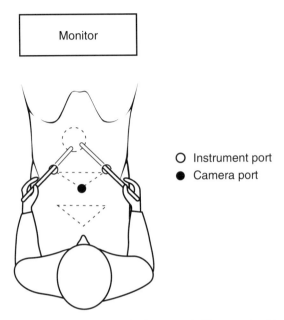

Fig. 4-1. Triangulation of ports. The coaxial alignment is illustrated with the surgeon, target tissue, suture line, and monitor all arranged along a straight path. Also shown are the positions of the surgeon's eyes and hands, as well as the viewing and two instrument ports.

The laparoscope and instrument ports should be placed in the same relative positions that these functions have in open surgery. That is, the camera should be midway between the two instrument ports, and the latter should be just forward of the surgeon's frontal plane *(center view triad)*. This mimics the normal relationship between the eyes and hands. The distance between the suturing ports should be approximately 20 cm. If the ports are closer or further apart, the surgeon may be able to suture, but it becomes more difficult. In this coaxial set-up, the surgeon, instrument ports, tissue, and video monitor should all be positioned along a straight line. When the surgeon attempts to suture in a different location, the three ports should be ideally shifted in unison to the new position.

The importance of port positioning is not only to provide the proper angle of access but also to provide a fulcrum for the instruments, which should be about halfway between the tip and the handle. That is, 50 percent of the instrument shaft should be inside the body cavity and 50 percent outside. This provides a 1:1 ratio of movement between the handle and tip. Port positioning is also discussed in Chapter 3.

For the right-handed surgeon, the suture line should be in the 11 o'clock to 5 o'clock position, and the stitches placed in a 2 o'clock to 8 o'clock direction. For the left-hander, the suture line should be 1 o'clock to 7 o'clock, and the stitches placed 10 o'clock to 4 o'clock.

Imaging System

Visual perception is a factor, because the operative field is viewed indirectly and from an altered perspective through a closed-circuit video system. Using current technology, a flat, two-dimensional image on a 14- to 19-inch monitor is provided that is subject to inadequate resolution and clarity.

The video system should consist of a three-chip camera and a high-resolution 19-inch monitor viewed from a distance of no more than 5 to 6 feet. Currently, the best equipment for suturing is a three-chip color camera and 19-inch monitor with a resolution of 700 horizontal lines, plus a digital image enhancer. For advanced laparoscopic surgery, second-rate imaging systems are unacceptable. Forthcoming systems incorporating stereoscopic vision hold promise for improved depth perception, which may be helpful to the beginner and to experienced surgeons in difficult situations. With experience, a high-quality two-dimensional image becomes more informative, especially with regard to spatial relationships, reference points, and interpretation of anatomy.

A 5- or 10-mm laparoscope with a Hopkins rod lens system is most commonly used for suturing. The lens must always be kept clean.

Visual Perception and Eye-Hand Coordination[6]

Magnification by the video system and the smallness of the operative field require a proportionate reduction of the speed and range of movement of the instruments to maintain control. The use of long-stemmed instruments pivoting at the abdominal wall adds to the challenge.

Frustration and fumbling are common in the novice. It is difficult at first to follow the trajectory of the two instrument tips, particularly when movements are fast and erratic. Even for experienced surgeons, the movements should be proportionately slower than in open surgery. The greater the magnification and the more the port position set-up deviates from the ideal, the more important this precept.

Although slowing down restores control, it also increases operating time. Suturing, which involves repetitious movements such as needle driving and knot tying, can be broken down into steps to facilitate learning. When suturing and knot tying movements are fully *choreographed*, precision increases and operating time decreases.

Random, nervous, and uncertain movements should be eliminated. Simply by eliminating unnecessary movements, even subtle ones such as regrasping tissue that falls away, a great deal of time is saved. This is another reason that the movements should be choreographed and then in practice kept as close as possible to the ideal.

Touch confirmation is a technique to enhance movement accuracy. It consists of touching the target structure to verify its location. In the process, spatial relationships become more apparent and are incorporated into visual memory. Touch confirmation helps improve accuracy and efficiency.

Suturing Instruments

Laparoscopic instruments for suturing have unique features. Because suturing and knot tying are two-handed tasks, the nondominant hand holds an assisting grasper, and the dominant hand the needle driver. Each has a specific role. The needle driver is primarily used to handle the needle and suture material, while a secondary task is to handle tissue. The grasper's main function is to hold the tissue and suture material and to assist in knot tying.

Although the handle and stems of the needle driver and grasper are similar, their jaws differ. The jaws of the needle holder are short and powerfully leveraged, maximizing grasping power. They should have a slight curve and a blunt point to facilitate looping the suture and for grasping the tissues and suture. The assisting grasper's narrow jaws should be more aggressively curved and pointed.

The suturing process requires both instruments to be rotated frequently, and thus the handle of the instrument should be cylindrical to allow a 360° rotation to be performed easily. Although this can be done with the traditional Roman scissors handle, it is considerably easier with a clam shell or rounded (coaxial) handle. As with needle holders for open surgery, a locking mechanism is desired to secure the grip on the needle. The shaft of the instrument should be about 33 cm for general use.

Suture Materials

The suture material is chosen to have attributes (i.e., absorbable vs. nonabsorbable, tensile strength, tissue reaction, etc.) primarily determined by the procedure. Nevertheless, other factors must be considered in laparoscopic surgery.

In regard to the needle, aside from wire strength and sharpness, visibility and curvature are important. The early pioneers used straight needles, because curved needles would not fit through the ports. Next came the ski needle, which was easy to pass through a port but also incorporated a curve at the tip for improved tissue pickup. Many laparoscopic surgeons, however, prefer the standard curved needle, because of the familiar and intuitive scooping motion involved in using it. Straight and ski needles are not practical for use in tight spaces because they tend to snag on tissues.

The thread should be visible, pliable, and hold knots securely. Silk has good pliability and is easy to work with, although it does have a tendency to fray when handled with instruments. Absorbable polyglactin or lactomer suture material is also easy to handle, but its lavender color may be a drawback against a dark background (e.g., blood and liver). Polyester, polygycolic acid, and polyglyconate sutures become less visible as they are stained with blood. The ideal suture material for laparoscopic surgery would have a vibrant, fluorescent (yellow, green, pink, blue, etc.) color.[7] ePTFE is better than most in this regard, because it is fluorescent white and resistant to staining.

Monofilament polypropylene, polydiaxanone, and nylon are strong, although their stiffness and excessive memory can make them more difficult to knot intracorporeally. Braided material holds a square knot securely but is unsuitable for an extracorporeal slip knot. For the latter, slippery monofilament material is better. If an intracorporeal square knot is tied with these sutures, the surgeon must remember to throw three to four hitches for adequate security.

Alternatives to Suturing

Although there are mechanical devices for approximating tissues edges and knotting, manually executed instrument suturing and knotting are still essential; suturing remains the most widely applicable means of tissue approximation.

The tension on the tissue may be varied much more than with mechanical devices, and in general, suturing is much cheaper than stapling. There are occasions when a considerable amount of time can be saved by using a mechanical stapling, ligating, or tissue anastomosis device. Even in these instances, however, suturing skills are needed, because the final stapled anastomosis often requires supplementation with a few sutures.

Training

Training programs should cover suturing, the square knot, surgeon's knot, and Aberdeen knot. The objectives should include time standards as follows: square knot, 30 seconds; placing a complete stitch, 90 seconds; performing an end-to-end or side-to-side anastomosis, less than 60 minutes. Practice should begin on inanimate materials and then progress to live animals.

Training should begin with exercises in a simulator (trainer box) using inanimate material. This provides an opportunity to become familiar with the equipment and the particulars of intracorporeal suturing and knot tying. Exercises typically begin with suturing a latex glove marked with two rows of dots on either side of a cut. Entrance and exit points should be targeted to avoid the development of bad habits.[9] Formal supervision is essential at the beginning.

The suture should be as short as possible and still able to accomplish the suturing task (the average is 6 to 8 inches). Longer sutures, although sometimes necessary for continuous suturing, easily become tangled. As with instrument tying in open surgery, the knot should always be placed at the distal end of the thread. The suturing area should be kept clear of slack suture.

Straight and ski needles can be inserted through a 5-mm port, but curved needles usually require a 10-mm cannula. By holding the thread 2 to 3 cm from the needle with the assisting grasper, it can be introduced through the port. By continuing to hold the thread at this point, the needle can be slowly lowered until the tip touches the tissue. The grasper can then be moved until the needle is oriented properly for placement in the needle holder. The appropriate grasping point is about two-thirds of the way from the tip of a ⅝ circle needle and half way from the tip of a half circle needle. If the needle is grasped at the correct point but is angled in the wrong direction, the tip can be hooked slightly on the tissue and, by pushing in one direction or another, can be pivoted into the proper position. To correct needle deflection (when the needle flips out of the proper position), the thread can be gently grasped about 1 cm behind the needle and pulled in a direction that restores the proper position. The grip on the needle driver must be loosened a little to allow this adjustment, but if loosened too much, the needle will be dropped altogether.

The needle should be held perpendicular to its plane for optimal security while advancing through the tissue. The needle point should puncture the tissue perpendicularly, and the needle should be driven through the tissue following the curve of the needle. Slow movements enhance precision.

Intracorporeal Knotting

Square Knot

The square knot (Fig. 4-2) is the standard for approximating tissues. While it is secure, it also can be tumbled into a slip knot[10] (two reversed half hitches), which allows adjustment of tension. In this form, it behaves as a jamming knot (i.e., when tightened against tension, it does not spontaneously loosen as an overhand knot does). Once secure, it can then be reoriented into the square knot configuration. Therefore, if it initially locks short of the intended position, a square knot does not usually have to be removed and replaced. It is best to place a third overhand throw on top of a square knot for additional security.

Surgeon's Knot

If tension develops as the tissues are approximated, the first overhand throw of a square knot may loosen. An overhand knot with two loops constitutes the "surgeon's knot," which resists tension more effectively (i.e., it is a reasonably good jamming knot). Another overhand throw on top of the surgeon's knot produces the equivalent of a square knot. The knot should be completed by placing the usual third overhand throw. Unlike a square knot, the knot formed by a surgeon's knot plus a second overhand throw cannot be adjusted. Therefore, if the tissue is too loosely approximated at this point, the knot must be cut and replaced. The surgeon's knot is the jamming knot of choice of many laparoscopic surgeons.

Other Less Common Knots

Granny Knot

The granny knot is composed of two half hitches placed in the same direction. The granny is theoretically less secure than a square knot, but in practice three overhand loops in a knot will suffice regardless of their orientation.

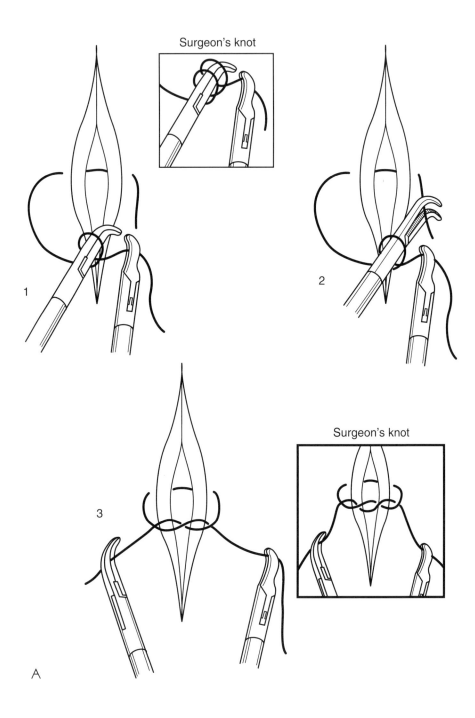

Surgeon's knot

1

2

3

Surgeon's knot

A

Fig. 4-2. Square knot and surgeon's knot. (**A**) First overhand flat knot. (1) Starting position. The right instrument reaches over to the left side of the field, grasps the long tail, and brings it back to the right, below the short tail. A C-loop is created, which must be in a horizontal plane or otherwise it is difficult to wrap the thread. When using monofilament material, the right instrument can rotate the thread counterclockwise until it lies flat against the tissue. With the long tail held by the right instrument, the left instrument is placed over the loop. The short tail should be long enough so that it will not be pulled out accidentally but not so long that its end is difficult to find. A large loop should be used to allow adequate excursion by both instruments when retrieving the short tail. The instruments should be moved slowly. Then, the right instrument is used to wrap the long tail around the stationary tip of the left instrument. The right instrument can be rotated forward (like turning a key), creating an arch in the suture, which facilitates this wrapping motion. The jaws of the instruments retrieving the short tail should be kept closed until near the tail and ready to grasp it. In the inset, the right instrument is shown wrapping the suture around the left instrument twice, to create a surgeon's knot. (2) Grasping the short tail. Both instruments should move toward the short tail. If they are not kept together, a tight noose forms around the instrument, making it difficult to open ("choking" the grasper). The short tail should be grasped as close to the end as possible to avoid creating an extra loop when pulling the suture. (3) Completing the first flat knot. The short tail should be pulled through the loop and adjusted so equal length is left. If the tail is too long, the end will be hard to find. The two instruments should then be pulled in opposite directions, parallel to the stitch. The left instrument drops the short tail, but the right instrument maintains its grasp on the long tail. The inset shows the results of a surgeon's knot that was created in Step 1. (*Figure continues.*)

1

2

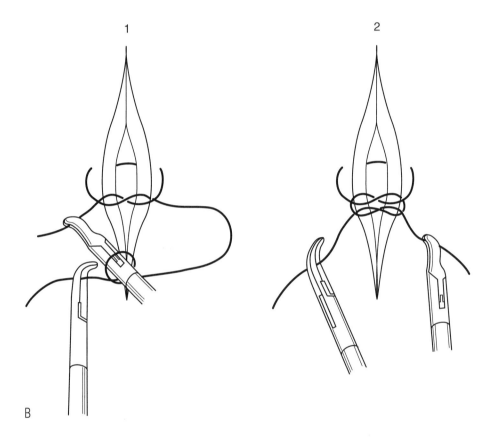

B

Fig. 4-2 (*Continued*). (**B**) Second opposing flat knot. (1) Creating the reversed C-loop and wrapping the thread and grasping the short tail. The right instrument is now brought to the left side of the field under the short tail and rotated clockwise 180° to create the reversed C loop. (Positioning and rotation can be done simultaneously.) The right instrument transfers the long tail to the left instrument. With the long tail now held by the left instrument, the right instrument is placed over the reversed C-loop. It is held steady while the left instrument wraps the long tail over and under the right instrument. Next, the tips of the right and left instruments are moved together toward the short tail, which is grasped with the right instrument. If difficulty is encountered, the long tail is regrasped so the thread held in the left hand is parallel to the instrument's jaws (as if the thread were an extension of the jaws). (2) Completing the second knot. The short tail should be pulled through the loop. The tails should be pulled in opposite directions, parallel to the stitch, with equal tension applied to both. The surgeon should check to make sure the knot is configured correctly (it should resemble the mathematical symbol for infinity). Adjusting the short tail: If possible, the instruments should pull the thread in one continuous movement until the knot is formed, rather than releasing the thread to regrasp it closer to the knot. The latter can be done afterward to tighten the knot. Completely forming the knot in one move may not be feasible, however, for knots in small spaces. (*Figure continues.*)

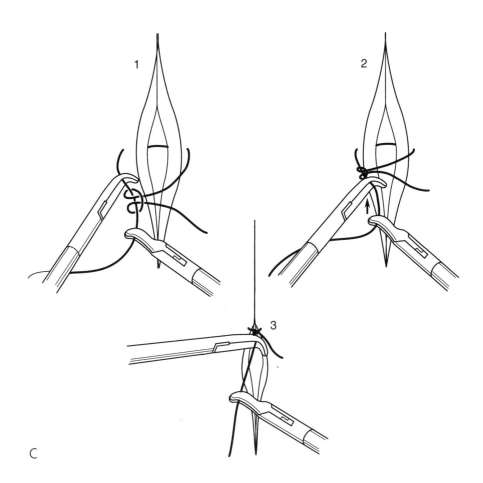

C

Fig. 4-2 (*Continued*). (**C**) Slip knot (for the square knot only). (1) Starting position and pulling. To convert the square knot (locking configuration) to a slip knot (sliding configuration), both instruments must grasp the suture on the same side. Either the right or left side can be used. One instrument grasps the thread outside the knot and the other in the suture loop (between the knot and the tissue). Left and right instruments pull in opposite directions (perpendicular to the stitch). Depending on how tight the knot is in the first place, a snapping or popping sensation can often be felt, and the short tail can be observed to flip up suddenly. The knot now resembles a double eyelet or pretzel. If the conversion does not occur after a couple of attempts, the same maneuver may be tried on the other side of the knot. Conversion is easier on monofilament than on braided suture. This maneuver is very different for a surgeon's knot. (2) Pushing the slip knot. The right instrument maintains its grasp on the tail and pulls tautly. The left instrument slides on this tail, pushing the knot closer to the tissue. If the knot does not slide, there are two things to check: (a) The square knot was not converted to a half hitch configuration or (b) the instrument pushing the knot is actually grasping or (squeezing) the knot or thread instead of sliding on it. The surgeon may try sliding the instrument along the suture tail before attempting to push the knot again. (3) Cinching down. The slip knot is cinched down until the tissue edges have been approximated to the desired tension. The knot should be recentered and the tension rechecked. If the stitch is still loose, further cinching (knot pushing) may be needed. The slip knot must be reconverted to a square knot (locking configuration) before additional overhand throws are made. Right and left instruments regrasp the tails on their respective sides in opposing directions, parallel to the stitch in the same way as when the square knot was originally tied. The slip knot has now been reconverted to a locked square knot. An additional overhand knot should be placed on top.

Twist Knot

The twist knot was promoted because it supposedly avoids the complex movements required in tying a square knot. The long tail is grasped by the needle driver and rotated three or more times around its axis. Then the short tail is pulled through this coil and pulled tight to create a knot (e.g., similar in design to a surgeon's knot). Although it seems simple, the twist knot requires considerable skill.

Lasso Knot

In the lasso knot, the end of the suture is looped and tied approximately 3 to 5 mm from the end, either as a permanent or slip knot. As the needle is driven through the tissue, it is passed through the loop, so when the thread is pulled, the tissue edges are brought together. The slip knot version is preferred, because the loop can be tightened. It is critical, however, to orient the slip knot correctly, because the loop will unravel if created with the mirror image orientation.

Prelooped Suture

This "prelooped" suture is introduced into the surgical field through a port. The needle is driven through the entrance and exit points and then passed through the pretied suture loop, secured by the tip of the applicator. Then the thread is held taut and the applicator handle is pushed, tightening the loop and creating the knot. The threads are then cut. These commercially available products, though helpful, do not preclude the need for knotting skills.

Performing a Continuous Suture

When performing a continuous suture, it is crucial to maintain tension on the tissue as the suture line is created. Re-adjusting the suture afterward can be very difficult. The simplest method of maintaining tension is to have an assistant follow the suture line by grasping the most recent stitch. It is also possible for the surgeon to follow himself or herself by using a suture grasper to maintain tension, but this makes placing the next stitch more difficult. Another technique to maintain tension is to lock the suture line after every three to four sutures.

In practice, especially when leakage of bowel contents is a concern, it may be safer to place a row of interrupted sutures rather than a continuous suture, especially for the inexperienced surgeon.

The end of a continuous suture line can be secured in several ways. The best way is to place a separate interrupted suture at the end of the continuous one and then to tie the end of the continuous suture to one tail of the interrupted suture. This method allows tension on the continuous suture to be adjusted appropriately. Another is to loosen the last loop and use it as the short tail for a square knot. A third method is the Aberdeen knot (Fig. 4-3), also known as the crochet, French, or western knot, which also requires loosening the last loop. Although the Aberdeen knot requires minimal rotation of the instrument, it may be difficult to execute properly, without losing tension on the suture line.

Extracorporeal Knotting

Extracorporeal knots are useful when the intracorporeal space is too tight for tying. They work best with slippery monofilament suture materials, because knots tied with braided suture have a tendency to lock too soon. The most common knot tied extracorporeally is a square knot, which is slipped into position in its tumbled half-hitch orientation and then reconfigured into a square knot.

Sliding Knot

In the sliding knot, a half-hitch is tied, and this is pushed down through the port with a knot pusher into the appropriate position. Then the second, third, and fourth overhand knots are tied and pushed down on top of each other. Although relatively simple, this is cumbersome, minimizes control of the stitch, and may place excessive tension on the tissues.

Roeder Knot

The Roeder knot (Fig. 4-4) is the ultimate in jamming knots. Pretied ligatures available commercially generally use this knot, which when pushed into position is secure enough that extra loops are usually unnecessary.

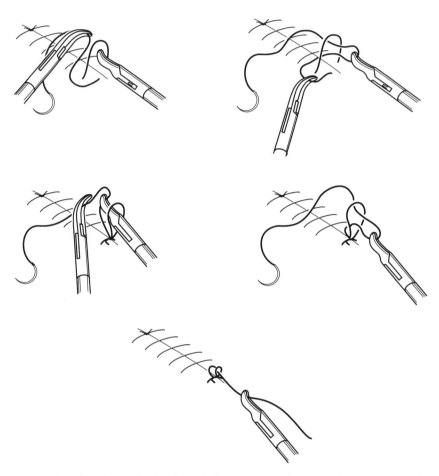

Fig. 4-3. Aberdeen knot. The last loop is loosened, and the needle driver is used to reach through this loop to grasp the long tail 5 to 10 mm from its exit from the tissue, pulling it through and cinching down the original loop (to the desired location and tension) and creating a new loop. This loop is then shortened, and the process is repeated two more times. After the third loop is created, the full suture, including the needle, is pulled through it, forming a permanent knot. It is crucial that the first cinch create the appropriate amount of tension on the tissues, because the knot cannot be adjusted after the second or subsequent loops are made. However, it can be unraveled and started again if the full suture, with needle, has not yet been pulled through.

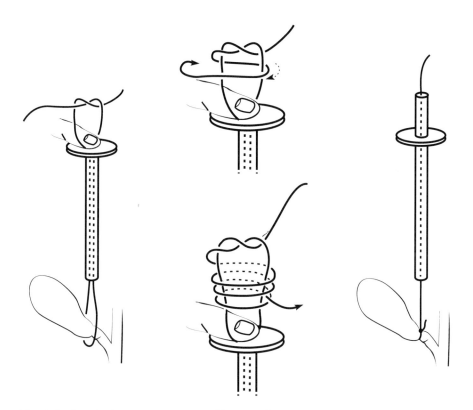

Fig. 4-4. Roeder knot (extracorporeal knot). A long suture is introduced intracorporeally, leaving the end outside the port. The needle is driven through the tissue and brought out the same port. An overhand flat knot is then tied. One end is then wrapped (coiled) around the main lead several times and pulled back through the last loop and tightened. Then, using a knot pusher with one hand and holding the lead thread with the other, the knot is pushed down to the desired position.

REFERENCES

1. Guthrie CC: Blood Vessel Surgery and Its Application: a Reprint. U Pittsburgh, Pittsburgh, 1959
2. Semm K: Tissue-puncher and loop-ligation: new aides for surgical therapeutic pelviscopy (laparoscopy): endoscopic intraabdominal surgery. Endoscopy 10:119, 1978
3. Reich H: Laparoscopic reversal of sterilization (abstract). Presented at the Second World Congress of Gynecologic Endoscopy, Flairemont-Ferrand, France, June 5–8, 1989

4. Estes JM, Szabo Z, Harrison MR: Techniques for in utero endoscopic surgery—a new approach for fetal intervention. Surg Endosc 6:215, 1992
5. Szabo Z. Berci G: Extracorporeal and intracorporeal knotting and suturing technique. p. 367. In Berci G (ed): GI Endoscopy Clinics of North America. WB Saunders, Philadelphia, 1993
6. Szabo Z. Laparoscopic suturing and tissue approximation. p. 141. In Hunter JG, Sackier JM (eds): Minimally Invasive Surgery. McGraw-Hill, New York, 1993
7. Bowyer DW, Moran ME, Szabo Z: Laparoscopic suturing in urology: a model for vesicourethral anastomosis following radical prostatectomy. Min Invas Ther 4:165, 1992
8. Wolfe BM, Szabo Z, Moran ME et al: Training for minimally invasive surgery: need for surgical skills. Surg Endosc 7:93, 1993
9. Szabo Z, Patton GW: Microsurgical Laparoscopy. p. 207. In Behrman SJ, Patton GW, Holtz G (eds): Progress in Infertility. 4th Ed. Little, Brown, Boston, 1993
10. Szabo Z, Stellini L, Rose EH et al: Slip-knot suspension technique: a fail-safe microanastomosis technique for small caliber vessels. Microsurg 13:100, 1992

5

▶ Operating Room Set-Up

C. Stirling
S. Bhoyrul

SETTING UP AN OPERATING ROOM APPROPRIATELY IS ESSENTIAL TO THE success of a laparoscopic procedure. In addition to the requirements for an open procedure, the operating room staff must be familiar with the unique features of the laparoscopic patient, laparoscopic operating room, and laparoscopic procedure. These factors will affect checking in a patient, verification of the operation, selection of instruments, equipment location in the room, preoperative checks for special equipment, and selection and positioning of the operating room table. In this relatively new field, the emphasis is on teamwork, good communication, and support. The team consists of the surgeon, anesthesiologists, nurses, technicians, orderlies, instrument processing personnel, and clerical staff. Some hospitals may have operating rooms dedicated to laparoscopic surgery, while in others, the room may have to be set up for each case using mobile equipment (usually on a cart). Regardless of the time of day, surgeons and administrators must realize that these factors add to the time and manpower required for a laparoscopic case.

This chapter covers issues unique to a laparoscopic operating room and emphasizes the information that the surgeons must communicate to the other members of the operating room team.

The members of the operating room team work simultaneously. Their different functions consist of the preoperative check-in of the patient, gathering the special equipment and supplies, organizing the operating room, and performing a preoperative check to make sure the equipment is in working order. The following information is required by the operating room staff as they work to prepare the patient and room for a laparoscopic procedure. The information can be conveniently organized into checklists as shown below.

Laparoscopic Equipment

The equipment and supplies needed will be determined by the kind of procedure and the surgeon's preferences, which should be conveyed to the operating room staff before the patient enters the suite. While the circulating nurse and anesthesiologist prepare the patient, other operating room staff assemble the items listed in Checklist 2.

Operating Room Set-Up

The positioning of the equipment in the operating room should be established before the patient enters the room.

Checklist 1: Preoperative Check-in of the Laparoscopic Patient

1. Collect the relevant patient information as for an open surgical case.
2. Obtain consent.
   a. Verify the kind of laparoscopic procedure planned (i.e., diagnostic laparoscopy followed by a laparotomy or a complete laparoscopic procedure) The consent should always include possible conversion to open surgery.
   b. Determine the patient's understanding of what surgical procedure will be performed.
3. Surgical history: In particular, assess whether the patient has had previous abdominal surgery. If so, a Hasson cannula (or similar device) should be made available, allowing the surgeon access the abdominal cavity using the open technique.

Checklist 2: Laparoscopic Equipment and Supplies

1. Sterile instruments: The instruments should be individualized to the procedure and personal preferences of the surgeon. An appropriate set of instruments to convert the laparoscopic case to open should be available from the start. The following equipment is common to nearly all laparoscopic procedures:
   a. Rigid laparoscopes: 10 mm, both in 0° and 30° versions. A 5-mm scope is often useful.
   b. Video camera: The highest quality (the three-chip) camera should be used. If not available, the surgeon should be informed before the start of the case, because an alternative unit may not be acceptable, and the case may have to be postponed.
   c. Fiber-optic light cord with connecting piece for the laparoscope that will be used.
   d. Veress needle and sterile insufflation tubing.
   e. Trocar-cannula devices of the size and specification appropriate for the case. Reducer valves and fascial threads.
   f. Antifogging solutions and/or laparoscope warmer.
   g. Suction-irrigation equipment with bag of irrigant fluid (usually heparinized saline).
2. Imaging equipment: The laparoscopic equipment cart should contain the following equipment.
   a. Main television monitor (preferably 19")
   b. Camera console box
   c. Light source
   d. Video cassette recorder
   e. Accessory television monitor (on another cart)
   f. Specialized recording equipment (e.g., slide maker and video printer)
3. Insufflator: This is also usually on the equipment cart. A carbon dioxide gas tank should be connected to the inlet

(Continues.)

valve of the insufflator, and a reserve gas tank should be available. The surgeon should know the maximum flow capability of the insufflator.

4. Cautery unit: In addition to an electrosurgical generator, which is the same as that used in an open case, a laparoscopic handset, with the ability to mount different electrodes (e.g., hook electrode and spatula) is also usually required. The incorporation of suction-irrigation into the electrode is often preferred. Sterile connecting cable must be available, and a cable to connect the hand-held instruments to an electrosurgical generator should also be available. If the surgeon wishes to use bipolar instruments, these should be available, but it is usually necessary to have a separate bipolar generator.

5. Radiographic equipment (if needed): The best equipment for cholangiograms is a digital video fluoroscopy unit with a C-arm.

6. Positioning devices such as a laparoscopic Bookwalter retractor, Leonard arm, or other mechanical assisting device may be required.

7. Operating room table of choice (as determined by the proposed patient positioning and procedure—see below).

8. Sequential compression stockings are used on the majority of laparoscopic patients. Some form of deep venous thrombosis prophylaxis is required for nearly all laparoscopic procedures.

When positioning the monitors, the direction in which the surgeon will be operating should be considered (see Ch. 3 for details of coaxial set-up). The surgeon, depending on the procedure, stands to the right or left of the patient or between the patient's legs and directs his attention toward the patient's upper or lower body. Thus, the main television monitor should be positioned in the most direct line of vision for the surgeon, while the secondary monitor should be in line with the assisting surgeon (usually on the side opposite the main monitor).

The main television monitor cabinet contains most of the electronic equipment used during the endoscopic procedure. Mounting the television monitor on a swivel extension arm from the top of the video cabinet simplifies its positioning over the patient's head. The insufflator should be located high in the cabinet, so the surgeon can see the display of intra-abdominal pressure and flow rates. The other equipment kept in the main cart usually consists of the camera console box, light source, and video recorder as well as any specialized imaging or recording equipment (e.g., mixers, printers, or slide makers). A second cart, if available, is convenient to mount the accessory monitor and store unopened disposable equipment, such as clip appliers and staplers. This system should be easy to move because it must be repositioned often to keep in line with the assistant surgeon. If a second insufflator is required, it can be put on this ancillary cart.

The cautery unit is best located next to the secondary monitor. It should be compatible with both disposable and reusable instruments and feature both hand and foot controls.

Other specialized pieces of equipment such as ultrasonic cutting devices or argon beam coagulators may be needed. For cholangiograms, the C-arm should approach the field from the patient's right, while a mobile lead shield is used to protect the surgeon on the opposite side. The surgeon usually injects the contrast media during the fluoroscopy.

Figure 5-1 depicts the typical operating room set-up for upper abdominal and thoracoscopic procedures, and Figure 5-2 shows the set-up for pelvic procedures.

The three most common patient positions are supine (with or without fluoroscopy capabilities), low lithotomy (often with the surgeon standing between the patient's legs), and right or left lateral decubitus (usually for thoracoscopic procedures). All three require a different operating room table set-up and positioning devices and are considered separately in the following section.

Supine Set-Up With Fluoroscopy

The operating room table is positioned to allow the C-arm to embrace the tabletop freely without obstruction (Fig. 5-3). Either a portable fluoroscopy tabletop extension with a radiolucent armboard (for extending the patient's left arm if desired by the anesthestist) or a radiolucent operating room table should be used. If the radiolucent operating room table is used, the tabletop or tabletop configuration should be reversed so the supporting pedestal does

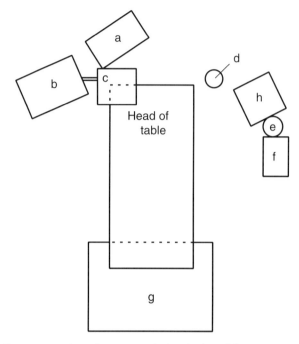

Fig. 5-1. Operating room set-up for upper abdominal and thoracoscopic procedures. a, Anesthesia machine; b, main video system cabinet; c, main video monitor;
d, IV pole; e, suction canister; f, cautery unit; g, overhead (Gerhardt) instrument
table; h, secondary video monitor.

not interfere with the fluoroscope arm (a regular armboard may be attached
to the table railing on the patient's left). (Fig. 5-4).

Some tabletop warming blankets are radiolucent and others are not. If a
warming blanket is used during a laparoscopic procedure requiring radiographic study, turning the circulation of the unit off during the study gives a
better image.

The type of fluoroscopy unit available varies between institutions (because it
is rarely purchased just for laparoscopic surgery). If a choice is available, the
highest resolution unit with the ability to produce a hard-copy film is desired.

Supine Set-Up Without Fluoroscopy

If fluoroscopy is not essential, a routine operating table set-up can be used. To
be prepared for the potential need of an intra-operative flat plate radiograph,

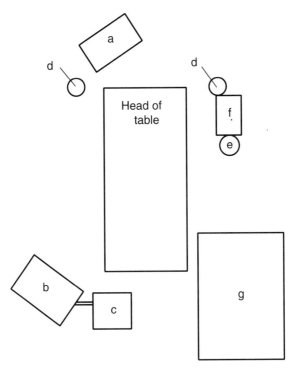

Fig. 5-2. Operating room set-up for pelvic laparoscopic procedures. a, Anesthesia machine; b, main video system cabinet; c, main video monitor; d, IV pole; e, suction canister; f, cautery unit; g, overhead (Gerhardt) instrument table or back table, situated to the side of the operating table. The secondary video monitor is optional and is not pictured.

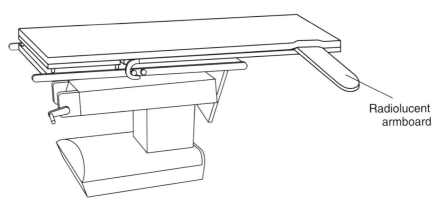

Fig. 5-3. Supine positioning with fluoroscopy tabletop attachment. A C-arm tabletop is shown with the table top turned 180° and the foot of the table lowered. The radiolucent armboard is shown slid under the mattress.

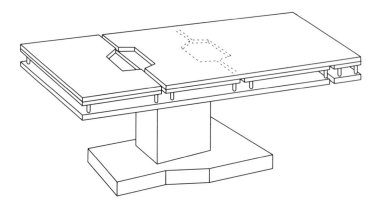

Fig. 5-4. Supine set-up with radiolucent table. The head extension has been placed at the foot of the table and the table reversed. A regular armboard (not shown) may be attached to the left table side rail.

the radiolucent tunnels for the operating room tables should remain in place for the laparoscopic procedure.

Low Lithotomy Set-Up

The low lithotomy set-up (Fig. 5-5) is commonly used for procedures in the pelvis and is similar, from a set-up point of view, to the steep reverse Trendelenburg position used for operating on the upper gastrointestinal (GI) tract. The Allen type of low lithotomy stirrups with table attachments are the leg holders of choice in this position. Padding should be available, as well as straps to secure the lower legs securely in the boot of the holders.

A mattress pad for the upper portion of the table can be altered by attaching a strip of wide Velcro to the lower half of the mattress lengthwise at the midline. The other half of the Velcro is attached to a large upper body vacuum bean bag (e.g., Vac-Pak). The bean bag is then attached to the mattress, using the Velcro strips, with enough length extending beyond the break in the table to allow the bag to be brought up around the patient's buttocks. Once the patient's legs are positioned in the stirrups, the bean bag is shaped into a shallow saddle, and the air is evacuated. This helps keep the patient from slipping down the table when in a steep reverse Trendelenburg position. A sheet is used to cover the bean bag and the upper portion of the mattress (under

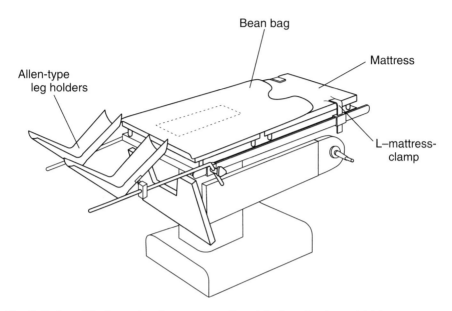

Bean bag

Mattress

Allen-type
leg holders

L–mattress-
clamp

Fig. 5-5. Low lithotomy (or steep reverse Trendelenburg) set-up. A Velcro vacuum bean bag is positioned atop the mattress, and the mattress and bean bag are secured to the table with L–mattress-clamps. Allen-type leg holders and table attachments are in place.

the patient). The sheet and mattress are doubly secured to the bed by an L–mattress-clamp at the head of the table (Fig. 5-5).

Lateral Decubitus Set-Up

The lateral decubitus set-up (Fig. 5-6) is the position commonly used for adrenalectomy, splenectomy, and thoracoscopic procedures. A right lateral or left lateral position may be used, depending on the side on which the procedure is to be performed (the operative side should point upward).

A large upper body vacuum type of bean bag with an axillary roll is used to stabilize the patient. The dependent arm may be placed on an armboard attached to the table railing, while the upper arm is supported on an "airplane" type of armrest (some are easier to attach and position than others). Ample blankets or pillows are used to support the thigh, with additional padding for the lateral aspects of the lower leg. A commercially produced sponge "donut" headrest is used to maintain head alignment.

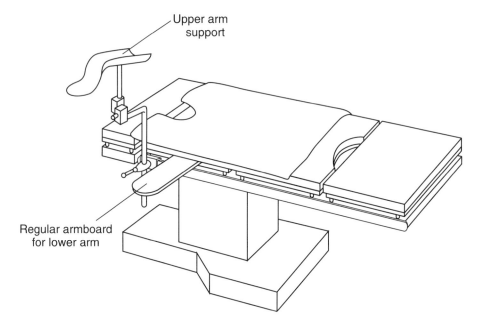

Fig. 5-6. Lateral decubitus set-up: routine set-up with vacuum bean bag atop the mattress. A support for the upper arm is in place in addition to the armboard for the lower arm. Extra blankets and padding are also required.

Once all the equipment is in the room, a preoperative check must be performed, as suggested in the following list:

Checklist 3: Preoperative Equipment Check

1. Television monitors
   a. Connect the main and accessory monitors with their signal input cables, which originate from the signal output ports on the back of the camera console box. These cables may pass directly from the camera box to the monitor, or the signal may be transmitted first to a video recorder or from the main monitor to the accessory monitor. Whichever type of signal is trans-
   (Continues.)

mitted (composite, Y/C, or RGB—see Ch. 2 for details) should be selected on the switch in front of the monitor.

   b. Connect the power plug for the main and accessory monitor carts to the electrical outlets.

   c. Turn both monitors on, and examine the monitors to adjust the appropriate color controls and termination switch on the secondary monitor. Failure to terminate the signal will result in a ghost image (see Ch. 2 for explanation).

2. Camera console box: Turn the unit on. The different brands of cameras display different images on the monitor during this phase. Some show color bars continuously, whereas others may only flash the color bars temporarily, then some words such as "head error," and then a blank screen. Whatever is the norm for the camera being used should be seen on both monitors. If the camera head is available at this point, connect the cable to the control box, and focus the image. Because the head is most often kept sterile, this step is usually performed before sterilization or after the surgeon has prepared and draped the field.

3. Video recorder: Turn the video recorder on. If the signal from the camera console box is transmitted first to the video recorder and then to the monitor, the recorder will have to be turned on before an image appears.

4. Insufflator: Turn the insufflator on. Check the carbon dioxide volume and confirm that it is adequate (as indicated by a dial on the insufflator). Set the maximum intra-abdominal pressure to 14 mmHg and the flow rate to 1 L/min or "low". Turn the gas flow on to confirm that gas actually flows from the system, and then partially occlude the outflow to test the audible alarm that sounds when the intra-abdominal pressure exceeds the

(Continues.)

desired setting. Once this test is done, the display showing the total volume of gas used should be reset to zero.

5. Turn on and test any additional special equipment on
the video cart that may be used during the case.

6. Check the cautery unit, ground pad availability, and set
the desired settings, if known, at this time.

7. Connect the vacuum pump to the suction canister and
position it near the cautery unit, because this will facilitate the use of a combined cautery-suction-irrigation
unit.

8. Prepare the heparinized irrigation commonly used
(usually 5000 U of heparin in 1000 ml of normal saline
or lactated Ringer solution), and label the additives in
the solution. Put the solution in a pressure bag and sus-
pend it from an intravenous (IV) pole.

9. Double-check the laparoscopic instruments and supplies for completeness and surgeon preference. Have
the instruments for an emergency laparotomy sterile
and available in the room.

10. Double-check the operating table set-up before bringing the patient into the room. Check the positioning
equipment.

11. Have antithromboembolic stockings (TED hose) and
compression stockings and machine available.

12. The patient may be brought into the operating room
only after all the above-mentioned checks have been
successfully completed, or with the agreement of the
surgeon if any check is incomplete or fails. This routine
should avoid the unacceptable situation where a laparoscopic case has to be abandoned because of "instrument
failure."

Conclusion

When every member of the surgical team works together and is familiar with the equipment and instruments available in their operating room, laparoscopic procedures can proceed smoothly and with the best chances of success. Laparoscopic surgery is growing more popular but also more complex, especially with regard to instrumentation, so it is important to stay current, maintain all instruments and equipment, and follow established safety measures and checklists.

Troubleshooting

Q.-Y. Duh

LAPAROSCOPIC OPERATIONS REQUIRE NEW SURGICAL INSTRUMENTS AND techniques. The surgeon must learn to view the anatomy indirectly (via a laparoscope and video monitor) and to manipulate the tissues remotely with less freedom than in open procedures. To perform laparoscopic operations successfully and with the least frustration, the surgeon and surgical team need to understand how the laparoscopic equipment works, and they must be able to diagnose, manage, and prevent the most common technical problems.

This chapter covers the most frequent technical problems in laparoscopic operations and discusses their management and prevention. Because only the surgeon knows the intended results in detail, the surgeon should know how to troubleshoot the problems. One cannot rely solely on operating room nurses or technicians, whose knowledge varies greatly, especially on evenings and weekends.

The problems in laparoscopic procedures are related to (1) establishing or maintaining the pneumoperitoneum, (2) exposure of anatomy, (3) video imaging, (4) hemorrhage, and (5) instrument failure. A systematic approach is the key to successful troubleshooting.

Problems in Establishing or Maintaining a Pneumoperitoneum

Problem: Cannot Establish the Pneumoperitoneum (Table 6-1)

The insufflator readings should be checked when a Veress needle is being used to establish the pneumoperitoneum. Early high-pressure and low-

Table 6-1. Problems in Establishing the Pneumoperitoneum: Early High Pressure and Low Flow Indicate Carbon Dioxide Flow Is Obstructed

Problem	Management
Veress needle too short	Use a longer Veress needle
Heavy abdominal wall	Lift the abdominal wall with towel clips
Needle in viscera	Remove needle, inspect viscera
Prior multiple abdominal incisions	Place trocar by the open technique
Distended small bowel or colon	

flow readings before the pneumoperitoneum is established are usually caused by positioning the needle tip outside of the free intra-abdominal space (see Ch. 3 for the proper technique of Veress needle insertion). This problem is more likely to occur in obese patients.

In an obese patient, the abdominal wall may be too thick for the Veress needle to penetrate the peritoneum. The needle may be in the abdominal wall or the preperitoneal space. Creation of a pneumo-*pre*peritoneum is especially common in the lower abdomen, and it makes trocar placement more difficult. A longer Veress needle should be used in markedly obese patients, or the needle should be inserted with a more perpendicular orientation than usual.

The presence of a pneumo-preperitoneum can be recognized after the trocar is placed because the transparent peritoneum can be seen through the scope. If the bowel appears to move freely beneath the peritoneum, the peritoneum can be grasped and incised to enter the intra-abdominal space.

Another problem in obese patients is created by the weight of the heavy abdominal wall, which can result in a pressure of 15 cmH$_2$O being reached before the peritoneal cavity is fully insufflated. This can be diagnosed and managed by lifting the abdominal wall with towel clips to relieve the pressure. Placing the patient in the head-up–feet-down position or the lateral decubitus position also allows the panniculus to fall away and may lessen intra-abdominal pressure. The lateral decubitus position may provide less intra-abdominal space, however, if the panniculus is supported too firmly (e.g., by a beanbag).

Early high pressure and low flow in the absence of a good pneumoperitoneum can also occur if the needle is inserted into a solid organ, such as the liver or spleen. In rare instances, this may cause a carbon dioxide embolism (see Ch. 8) and even cardiac arrest. If the needle is inserted into the intestine, insufflation will lead to uneven distension of the abdomen. These problems should be rare if the Veress needle is inserted properly and no blood or bowel contents were aspirated initially (see Ch. 3). The viscera should be inspected at the beginning of any laparoscopic procedure to make sure they have not been injured by the Veress needle or a trocar.

If a pneumoperitoneum cannot be established with the Veress needle, or if the abdominal cavity is laced with numerous adhesions from previous operations or obscured by distended intestine, the open technique for trocar insertion should be used (see Ch. 3).

Problem: Cannot Maintain the Pneumoperitoneum (Table 6-2)

Inadequate pneumoperitoneum is a major cause of poor exposure during laparoscopic procedures (see the section *Problems in Exposure*). The cause can be quickly determined by knowing the pressure and flow of the insuf-

Table 6-2. Problems in Maintaining the Pneumoperitoneum

Problem	Management
1. Low pressure and low flow (insufficient carbon dioxide at the source)	Check carbon dioxide tank, use spare tank
	Check the valve connecting to the insufflator
	Check the pressure ceiling setting
2. High pressure and low flow (obstructed carbon dioxide flow)	Check the system for obstruction
Kinked or compressed tubing	Check tubing for obstruction, shorten tubing
Cannula valve	Turn the valve on
Cannula in the preperitoneal space	Reposition cannula, incise peritoneum
Large instrument	Connect the tubing to another cannula
Insufficient muscle relaxation Respiratory movement	Increase anesthesia
3. Low pressure and high flow carbon dioxide leakage in the system)	Check system for leakage
Leakage around the cannula site	Bubbling around the port site with saline
Cannula valve or reducer damaged	Use a new cannula or reducer
Reducer too large for instrument	Change reducer

flator and by following the flow of carbon dioxide through the system (Fig. 6-1).

Low Pressure and Low Flow (Insufficient Carbon Dioxide at the Source)

The gauge should be checked to make sure that the carbon dioxide tank is not empty and that the valve is open. The maximum pressure limit set on the insufflator should be checked; it should usually be about 15 mm Hg. A spare tank of carbon dioxide should always be available. Problems with insufficient carbon dioxide are avoidable by checking the system preoperatively.

High Pressure and Low Flow (Obstructed Carbon Dioxide Flow)

The tubing from the insufflator to the trocar should be checked, looking for kinks or compression by equipment. The surgeon should ensure that the maximum pressure setting is actually where intended.

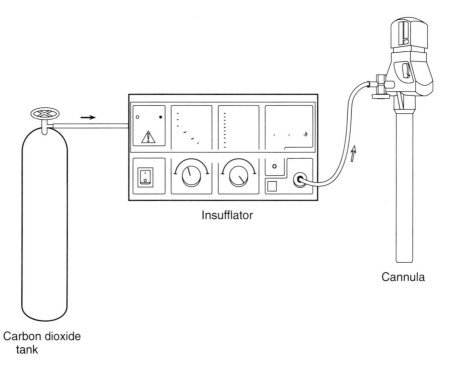

Insufflator

Cannula

Carbon dioxide
tank

Fig. 6-1. The flow of carbon dioxide from the gas tank to the patient. Any obstruction of or leakage from this system will lead to loss of pneumoperitoneum and poor exposure.

The obstruction may be at the trocar. The connection between the tubing and the trocar should be patent, and the gas inlet valve of the trocar should be in the open position. Obstruction at the tip of the trocar (e.g., if the tip has slipped back into the preperitoneal space or is against a viscus) can produce this problem. A large instrument can occasionally impede the flow of gas. Such problems can be diagnosed and solved by connecting the gas tubing to a different trocar.

Insufficient relaxation of the abdominal muscles or respiratory attempts by the patient are other common causes of a paradoxically high insufflator pressure. The diagnosis is usually easy to make visually once this possibility is thought of. The solution consists of establishing complete muscular relaxation. Laparoscopy under local anesthesia or limited regional anesthesia without abdominal relaxation inevitably involves a limited pneumoperitoneum, and it is more difficult than when general anesthesia is used with total muscle relaxation.

Low Pressure and High Flow (Leakage of Carbon Dioxide From the System)

The tubing from the insufflator to the trocar should be checked for leakage of carbon dioxide. The tubing near the trocar should be kinked by hand: The pressure should rise and the flow should stop if there is no leak in the tubing proximal to the kink. Most leakage of carbon dioxide occurs through or around the trocar. A leak around the trocar site (between the trocar and the skin) may be obvious, but it can be detected by the appearance of bubbles if the wound is covered with saline. The reducer or trocar valve may have been damaged by instruments, which can only be solved by replacing the defective unit. A common mistake is to use a reducer that is too large for the instrument (e.g., using a 5.5-mm reducer for a 4.5-mm instrument).

Problems in Exposure

Exposure is more difficult for laparoscopic than for open operations, because one cannot retract tissues by hand. Adequate exposure depends on the maximum use of gravity, the pneumoperitoneum, countertraction, and instruments.

Problem: Cannot See; Other Organs in the Way (Table 6-3)

Incorrect Patient Position

In general, the patient should be positioned with the area of interest elevated. This enlists gravity to help keep unwanted mobile organs, such as the small

Table 6-3. Problems in the Exposure of Anatomy

Problem	Management
Patient positioning	Use gravity to retract mobile organs
	Elevate the area of interest
Pneumoperitoneum	See Tables 6-1 and 6-2
Retraction technique	Proper direction
	Change grasping position as needed
	Operate with both hands
Positioning of instrument ports	Scope in the line of sight of surgeon
	Triangulate the ports for the scope
	and instrument
	Use angled scope

bowel, omentum, or transverse colon, out of the way. For inguinal hernia repair, the patient should be in a feet-up–head-down (Trendelenburg) position. For biliary and gastric operations, the patient should be head-up and feet-down. For appendectomy, the patient should be positioned right side up. When the area of interest changes during the operation (e.g., during mobilization of the colon), the patient should be repositioned to continue to use gravity to aid exposure. Another reason to elevate the area of dissection is to avoid pooling of blood, which could otherwise obscure the view.

Insufficient Pneumoperitoneum

See the section *Problems in Establishing or Maintaining a Pneumoperitoneum.*

Inappropriate Tissue Retraction

Proper countertraction is important for exposure. The direction is important. For example, lateral, not cephalad, traction should be applied to the infundibulum of the gall bladder to open Calot's triangle while the cystic duct is dissected. Medial and anterior traction is necessary to mobilize the colon.

In contrast to open operations, the range of retraction, especially during anterior retraction, may be limited by the abdominal wall and the position of the grasper. Tissues may have to be regrasped more often than in open procedures. In open adrenalectomy, a tag of connective tissue is usually used as a handle to retract the fragile adrenal gland. In laparoscopic adrenalectomy, however, multiple tags or a rim of connective tissue may be needed to allow frequent regrasping.

Whenever possible, the surgeon and the assistant should operate with both hands. In general, the nondominant hand can provide better retraction than can an assistant's hand. For prolonged stationary retraction, such as cephalad retraction on the fundus of the gall bladder in laparoscopic cholecystectomy, a fixed mechanical arm is superior to a human assistant.

Poor Positioning of Scope and Instruments

Proper positioning of the ports, the instruments, the scope, and the surgeon and assistants facilitates good exposure and avoids fatigue (see Ch. 3). Whenever possible, the scope should be directed along the line of sight of the surgeon and the assistant, which avoids operating with right and left reversed on the monitor, a very difficult situation even for experienced laparoscopic surgeons.

Proper positioning helps because the procedure occurs in a three-dimensional environment with only a two-dimensional view. The object of dissection, the port for the scope, and the port for the instruments should be arranged in a triangle of appropriate size (see Fig. 4-1). On the monitor, the instrument should appear to approach the object of dissection from a lateral direction so the full length of the instrument can be seen when the scope zooms out. Coaxial positioning of the instrument and the scope (e.g., as when using a scope with a dissecting channel, or with close positioning of the scope and the instrument ports) complicates the dissection because depth perception is poor. An angled scope is helpful if coaxial placement of the scope and the instrument cannot be avoided. The angled lens at the end of the scope allows the line of sight to be aligned optimally in relation to the instruments.

Problems With Video Images

The most common problem in laparoscopic surgery is a poor video image. There may be no image, poor-quality image, or extraneous interference on the monitor (Table 6-4).

Table 6-4. Problems With Video Images

Problem	Management
No image on the monitor	Check POWER ON status lights, power cords, plugs, power strip
	Match the selected input and output signals (Line A, Line B, Y-C, VTR) on the monitor
	Plug camera cable securely into the camera console box
	Disconnect the camera from the scope to see whether the scope is the problem
	Check the light source
	Line switch on the VCR should be on LINE or AUX and not CHANNEL
	Check the fuses in the camera control box and light source
Poor images on the monitor	
Dark grainy images are caused by insufficient light	Check the light source, take it off STANDBY
	Turn up the INTENSITY of the light source
	Turn up the GAIN in the camera box
	Turn up the BRIGHTNESS control on the monitor
Foggy image is caused by condensation	Apply defogging solution to the tip of scope
	Warm the scope; connect insufflator tubing to any cannula except the one for the laparoscope
	Avoid using liquid disinfectant
Blurred image is out of focus	Focus
Faded or inappropriate color	White balance
Interferences	
Jumpy images	Change damaged camera cable
Images with interference lines	Use a separate plug for the cautery unit
	Avoid crossing cables
Images with glare (ghosting)	Terminate video signal properly

Problem: No Image on the Monitor

To determine why there is no image on the monitor, first the path of the video signal should be traced from the monitor to its source (Fig. 6-2). The power should be on. The status lights on the equipment should be on if they are getting current. The power cords should be checked, and all components should be plugged in. Some devices may be plugged into a power strip with a separate switch that must be turned on.

The monitor usually has multiple signal inputs. The line input selected on the monitor (line A, line B, Y-C, VTR; see Ch. 2) must match how the video signal is received. To avoid recurrent problems, the routine line input selection should be labeled clearly and checked before the operation. The connectors of the camera cable should be securely plugged into the camera control box. Some connectors have metal pins, and others have flat metal strips; they need to be plugged in with proper orientation and good contact.

The camera head should be checked for damage. The scope should be disconnected from the camera head. If the camera head alone produces a good image, the problem is in the scope or its coupling to the camera. Another scope should be tried. Problems with illumination can be investigated by disconnecting the light cable from the scope or the light source to see that the light is on.

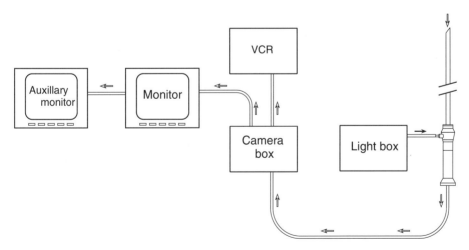

Fig. 6-2. The correct set-up for the imaging equipment and the path of the video signal from the laparoscope to the monitors.

Most systems include a video recorder (VCR) to record the procedure. The video signal from the camera control box is frequently routed through the VCR before it reaches the monitor. The VCR will have to be turned on, and the line switches set on LINE or AUX and not on CHANNEL number, to transmit the video signal properly to the monitor. Fuses in the camera control box and light source should be checked when the cause of the problem is localized to one of these devices.

Problem: Poor-Quality Image on the Monitor

Dark Grainy Image

A dark grainy image is usually caused by insufficient illumination. The surgeon should turn up the intensity of the light source, the gain in the camera box, or the brightness control on the monitor. The light source should be checked directly by disconnecting it from the light cable and the scope. Some light sources have a standby mode that produces a minimal amount of light to avoid overheating when full intensity is not needed. The light source should be switched off standby. The ends of the light cable should be inspected for debris and cleaned. The integrity of the optic fibers in the light cable can be checked by holding one end of the cable against the room light and inspecting the other end. Dark dots are caused by broken fibers. The cable should be replaced if more than 25 percent of the fibers are broken. The scope can be checked by looking through it directly; another scope can be used if doubt arises.

Foggy Image

Fogging is caused by condensation of water on the optics. If the image is clear until the scope is inside the patient, water is condensing on the lens at the end of the scope. Defogging solution (e.g., FRED or Betadine) should be applied, or the tip of the scope may be warmed by applying it to the liver. The end of the light cable is hot and could burn the patient. The end of the scope may also become hot, so it should not be defogged by touching it to the bowel. The best way to prevent fogging is to keep the scope at body temperature when it is outside the patient's abdomen. Connecting the insufflator tubing to any cannula except the one for the laparoscope will also reduce the likelihood of fogging.

Fogging can also occur between the eyepiece of the scope and the coupler or between the coupler and the camera head. The scope should be disconnected from the camera, and the eyepiece and the lens of the coupler should be dried. If fogging persists, the coupler should be disconnected from the camera head and both dried. The space between the coupler and the camera head is not sterile, so this should be done off the sterile area to avoid contamination, and the camera should be redraped using sterile technique afterward. Sterilizing the scope with liquid disinfectant such as Steris may allow water to condense between the coupler and the camera head. Sterilizing by gas prevents this problem. Condensation on the inside of the lens occurs only if there are cracks in the scope or the camera, in which case the defect will have to be repaired.

Blurred Image

A blurred image is caused by a scope that is out of focus. The focus ring on the coupler should be turned until the image becomes sharp. Each focus setting has a limited depth of field, just as with a 35-mm camera. Focus is lost faster while zooming in and out if the scope has been focused very close to the object. A blurred image is also caused by the problems described in the previous section.

Image With Faded or Inappropriate Color

Faded or inappropriate color is most commonly caused by an inappropriate color balance. The white balancing procedure should be repeated. If the camera and the control box have an automatic white balance, the automatic setting should be changed to manual and white balancing repeated. Damaged S-VHS connecting pins can cause inappropriate color (they may also cause a jumpy image; see below). A smear of color can occur if the connector between the camera cable and the control box is wet. The connector should be unplugged and both air dried. Inappropriate color can also be caused by the monitor being out of color adjustment. This is corrected by adjusting the color and hue controls of the monitor. A faster way is to press the reset button.

Problem: Interfering Images on the Monitor

Jumpy Images

Jumpy images are usually caused by a problem in the camera cable. A defective camera cable can be diagnosed by bending the cable along its length and watching to see if the picture jumps. The camera cable connecter should be securely seated in the camera control box. The BNC–S-VHS cable from the camera control box to the monitor should also be checked by bending it along its length.

Images With Interference Lines

Lines in the image are usually caused by electrical interference, most commonly from the electrocautery apparatus. The interference can be minimized by a proper set-up of the plugs and cables. The electrocautery unit should be plugged into a different power outlet from that used by the imaging equipment. The electrocautery cable and the camera cable should be draped off different sides of the table, and one should avoid crossing them. Insufficient insulation of the cable may be a cause of interference; the cable should be checked for damage.

Images With Glare (Ghosting)

Glare, or ghosting, is caused by improper video signal termination. The video signal is carried on a coaxial cable having a characteristic impedance of 75 ohms. The signal must be terminated at the end of the line of transmission; otherwise the signal will reflect and create a second, less distinct, image on the monitor. Most monitors are designed to receive and display the video image and to pass the video signal to another monitor if necessary. The last device in a video system with a series of units should be terminated by a 75-ohm resistor.

In some older monitors, glaring occurs because the monitor is not properly terminated. These monitors have a 75-ohm switch in the back, which should be turned on if the monitor is the last in a chain. When using a single monitor, its 75-ohm termination switch should be turned on; when using two monitors, the 75-ohm switch of the first monitor should be off, and the switch of the second monitor should be on. Although newer monitors terminate the signal automatically, glaring can still occur if a cable is connected to "lineout" but not connected to a second monitor. Plugging a cable into lineout tells the monitor that it is not the last device, and the signal will not be terminated. The solution is either to connect another monitor to the cable or to remove the cable from the first monitor.

Hemorrhage

Hemorrhage interferes with laparoscopic procedures more than open ones. The laparoscope tends to magnify the extent of bleeding; blood clots absorb light and decrease illumination; and blood splashed on the end of the scope decreases the amount of transmitted light and obscures the viewing lens.

When bleeding occurs, it is important not to panic, because the amount of bleeding is usually exaggerated by magnification. The surgeon should not clamp or cauterize blindly when the bleeding source cannot be seen, so as to avoid injury to important structures such as the common bile duct or ureter. A grasper should be used to gently tamponade the bleeding site. The area should then be cleared by suction and irrigation, and the exact source of bleeding identified. This should be done systematically, taking advantage of gravity, starting higher up and working downward where blood tends to pool. When the source is identified, it can then usually be managed by clips, endoloops, cautery, or sutures. Sometimes a 5-minute period of tamponade is alone sufficient to get substantial control, particularly with small vessels. An extra port may be added if needed for grasping or suction and irrigation. Small rolled-up sponges placed through a 10-mm trocar can be used to tamponade a bleeding vessel or to clear blood clots that absorb light. If the hemorrhage is severe, if a large vessel is injured, or if the site of hemorrhage cannot be identified, the abdomen should be opened. Any consideration of a transfusion indicates that bleeding is too severe for laparoscopic management.

Instrument Failure

Hand instruments can experience mechanical failure (e.g., a broken handle), so spare instruments should always be available. Cables, tubings, connectors, and other spare parts should be clearly labeled and stocked in the laparoscopic equipment cart. When the tip of an instrument is broken, the loose parts should be retrieved from the abdominal cavity and accounted for. A radiograph of the abdomen may be needed. If an instrument has become jammed in the open position and cannot be removed through the trocar, a heavy grasper should be inserted through another trocar and an attempt to close the instrument should be made. If unsuccessful, the trocar site will have to be enlarged, and the instrument removed along with the trocar.

The integrity of the insulation on instruments used with electrocautery should be checked before each procedure to prevent electrical injuries to the patient.

The surgeon should know the instruments to be used by their specific names (see Ch. 2 for the commonly used instruments). The surgeon should be familiar with new instruments before using them in the operating room. If an instrument is complex (e.g., a reusable stapler), the nurses and assistants should have in-service training before the operation.

Other Problems

Conversion to an Open Procedure

For any laparoscopic case, the surgeon should be prepared to convert to an open procedure. The indications include bleeding, poor exposure, and excessive difficulty with slow progress. Safety is the highest priority. If a laparoscopic case cannot be continued safely with a technical result equivalent to an open operation, it should be promptly converted. Therefore, the operating table should be set up appropriately, the extra equipment should be handy, and the anesthesiologist and scrub nurse should be prepared. Conversion to an open procedure should be considered good judgment rather than bad publicity.

Problems with Electrosurgery and Laser

For problems with electrosurgery or laser devices, see Chapter 2.

Problems with Trocar Site Closure

For problems with trocar site closure, see Chapter 3.

Conclusion

The surgeon should be familiar with the common problems that occur in laparoscopic surgery, which are usually related to establishing or maintaining the pneumoperitoneum, exposing the anatomy, video imaging, hemorrhage, and instrument failure. Knowing the possible causes of these problems and approaching them systematically will enable one to troubleshoot with minimal effort, so the surgeon can concentrate on the operation itself.

Acknowledgment

We thank Dave Stinebaugh of Karl Storz Endoscopy-America, Inc., and Allen Smoot of Stryker Endoscopy for their helpful input.

Suggested Readings

Gordon LA, Shapiro SJ, Daykhovsky L: Problem-solving in laparoscopic surgery. Surg Endoscopy 7:348, 1933

Hunter JG, Sackier JM: Minimally invasive surgery. p. 33. In Odell RC: Laparoscopic Electrosurgery. McGraw-Hill, New York, 1993

7

▶ Anesthetic Considerations

S. D. Kelley

Anesthetic Perspectives

THE RAPID EXPANSION OF LAPAROSCOPIC GENERAL SURGERY HAS BEEN accompanied by an increase in knowledge concerning the anesthetic aspects of minimally invasive surgery. Previous anesthetic experience in laparoscopic surgery had been gathered in brief gynecologic procedures performed principally in healthy young women. The introduction of laparoscopic cholecystectomy resulted in a reappraisal of the physiologic implications and anesthetic requirements for this type of surgery. In general, the physiologic changes observed during laparoscopic cholecystectomy are greater than those observed during gynecologic procedures and often occur in patients with significant coexisting disease. In a study of 101 patients undergoing laparoscopic cholecystectomy, the incidence of intraoperative and postoperative anesthesia morbidity (hypotension, desaturation, hypothermia, nausea and vomiting, excessive pain) was intermediate between gynecologic laparoscopy and open cholecystectomy.[1] Several recent review articles have helped provide an overview of the anesthetic issues involved in laparoscopic and thoracoscopic surgery.[2-5] The evolution of anesthetic techniques in the past 20 years has yielded anesthetic agents and adjuvants that provide a more rapid recovery from general anesthesia with a reduction in the incidence of anesthetic side effects. Use of appropriate anesthetic techniques and an understanding of the physiologic implications of the laparoscopic procedure should yield the greatest patient benefit from minimally invasive surgery.

Preoperative Considerations

The anesthetic plan should take into account coexisting illnesses. Patients presenting for laparoscopic general surgical procedures need to be evaluated preoperatively before anesthesia is administered. The goal is to identify medical and/or surgical conditions that require preoperative intervention or a specific modification of the anesthetic plan. Patients presenting for laparoscopic cholecystectomy may be healthy except for the cholelithiasis, but risk factors for cholelithiasis may have anesthetic implications. Obesity, for example, may increase esophageal reflux, or impair ventilatory mechanics. Elderly patients may have abnormal cardiopulmonary function and reserve. Patients with coronary artery disease or chronic obstructive pulmonary disease must be evaluated. The presence of heart or lung disease is not a contraindication to general anesthesia; the extent of disease, however, may modify the selection of anesthetic agents (to avoid tachycardia, maintain adequate blood pressure, etc.) or the use of intraoperative monitors (consideration for arterial and or pulmonary artery pressure monitoring).

Laboratory and diagnostic studies should be reviewed. Young, physically fit patients without other disease require few tests. Measurement of hemoglobin is appropriate in most women; tests of liver function and the clotting system are indicated in patients with bile duct obstruction or known hepatic disease. Electrocardiograms (ECGs) and chest radiographs should be limited to patients with cardiac or pulmonary disease or symptoms and those older than 50 years. Despite the infrequency of hemorrhagic complications during laparoscopy, a blood specimen should be sent to the blood bank for a type and screening (ABO/Rh blood type is determined, and the serum is screened for antibodies associated with transfusion reactions).

It is important to give instructions to the patient before surgery. One of the benefits of laparoscopic procedures is a shorter hospital stay. Patients are usually admitted on the morning of surgery and discharged within 12 to 24 hours. Surgery, anesthesia, and nursing teams must coordinate. The date and time of surgery should be confirmed, fasting guidelines made clear, and anticipated length of hospitalization discussed. Laparoscopic cholecystectomy may be done as a come-and-go procedure. In this situation, preoperative planning should include a discussion of transportation home following surgery and assistance at home that evening. The patient should be given a follow-up appointment and a way to contact the surgeon in case of questions or problems.

Anesthetic Management

Anesthetic Plan

The plan includes general anesthetic goals and specific goals related to the laparoscopic procedure. General goals include ensuring adequate analgesia, maintaining hemodynamic stability, and providing a smooth transition into the postoperative period. Specific goals include maximizing operative exposure and surgical conditions, anticipating physiologic changes, and maximizing the benefits of the minimally invasive approach.

Although laparoscopy can be performed with general, regional, or local anesthesia with sedation, there is no proof that any one of them is safest. Local or regional anesthesia is usually used for short diagnostic or therapeutic gynecologic procedures.[6] The difficulties in obtaining an adequate pneumoperitoneum has limited their use in general surgery. During regional anesthesia (epidural or spinal anesthesia), a high level of sensory, motor, and sympathetic denervation is required, which may be associated with hypotension. The patient may experience dyspnea as a result of the regional block, which could be exacerbated by the pneumoperitoneum and position changes. Finally, regional anesthesia may not be satisfactory if the chances of converting to an open procedure are high.

Regardless of the anesthetic technique, it is important to provide adequate abdominal wall relaxation. The carbon dioxide insufflator is usually set to keep intra-abdominal pressure at 15 mmHg. Adequate muscle relaxation increases abdominal wall compliance, allowing a larger space and better exposure, which is critical for safety. During a general anesthetic, a short- or intermediate-duration nondepolarizing muscle relaxant should be titrated to a peripheral nerve stimulator response. This will provide good relaxation and allow the block to be reversed rapidly at the end of the operation.

Several options are available for airway management. Oral endotracheal intubation is safe and facilitates controlled, positive pressure ventilation. A laryngeal mask airway has been used during brief procedures but is less desirable during longer ones.[7,8]

Some surgeons and patients have an impression that general anesthesia should be avoided if possible in high-risk patients with cardiovascular or pulmonary disease. In laparoscopic procedures, however, general anesthesia with controlled ventilation and intraoperative monitoring provide the greatest

Table 7-1. Hemodynamic Changes During Laparoscopic Cholecystectomy

Parameter	Baseline	Anesthesia	Head-Up	Insufflation
Mean arterial pressure, mmHg	96 ± 13	87 ± 3	71 ± 2	102 ± 5
Heart rate, bpm	79 ± 4	83 ± 4	76 ± 4	81 ± 5
Right atrial pressure, mmHg	8 ± 1	8 ± 1	5 ± 1	10 ± 1
Pulmonary capillary wedge pressure, mmHg	9 ± 1	9 ± 1	7 ± 1	14 ± 1
Cardiac index, $L \cdot min \cdot m^{-2}$	3.6 ± 0.1	2.7 ± 0.2	2.2 ± 0.2	2.4 ± 0.1
Systemic vascular resistance, $dynes \cdot s \cdot cm^{-5}$	1139 ± 49	1389 ± 108	1452 ± 111	1777 ± 146
Isoflurane, % inspired	—	.46 ± .03	.38 ± .04	1.02 ± .08

Values are mean ± SEM.
(Data from Joris et al.[11])

degree of hemodynamic and ventilatory stability.[9] The anesthesiologist and surgeon should communicate preoperatively regarding the management of patients with coexisting disease. This discussion should include the use of invasive monitoring and the possibility of admission to the intensive care unit following the procedure.

Intraoperative Physiologic Changes and Complications

The anesthesia team must be vigilant regarding potential complications and must anticipate physiologic changes known to be associated with laparoscopy.[10–12]

Important to the anesthesiologist is the hemodynamic effect of induction of anesthesia and the subsequent response to the surgical procedure. The anesthetic agents used, intravascular volume status, volume and pressure of insufflated carbon dioxide, and ventilatory management will affect the changes. Joris and colleagues[11] measured hemodynamic changes in 15 healthy, nonobese patients who underwent laparoscopic cholecystectomy with a standard anesthetic regimen and invasive hemodynamic monitoring. Hemodynamic changes in response to the induction of anesthesia, the reverse Trendelenburg position, and the pneumoperitoneum are summarized in Table

7-1. Among the most notable events was the acute response to creation of the pneumoperitoneum. Increases in mean arterial pressure, central venous pressure (CVP), pulmonary capillary wedge pressure (PCWP), and systemic vascular resistance (SVR) were associated with a decreased cardiac index. Despite the increase in measures of filling pressure (CVP, PCWP), true intraventricular filling volumes may have decreased. With creation of the pneumoperitoneum, intrathoracic pressure increased by approximately 9 mmHg, so that the net change in true filling pressure (i.e., CVP − intrathoracic pressure) decreased during the period of pneumoperitoneum. The increase in SVR accounts for the elevation in mean arterial pressure despite the reduction in cardiac index, as has been noted in other studies. One hypothesis states that the pneumoperitoneum and compression of the abdominal aorta are responsible for the increase in SVR. Other evidence suggests that creation of the pneumoperitoneum or surgical stimulation releases humoral mediators (e.g., vasopressin, prostaglandins, catecholamines, and the renin-angiotensin system), which produce the observed changes in SVR. Initial increases in SVR following creation of the pneumoperitoneum may be modified by the increasing concentration of isoflurane, an inhalation anesthetic with known vasodilation properties. Another investigation that used transesophageal echocardiography demonstrated preservation of left ventricular ejection fraction during laparoscopic cholecystectomy.[13] In this study, the pneumoperitoneum resulted in increases in systemic blood pressure and left ventricular end-systolic wall stress; head-up positioning also decreased the end-diastolic ventricular volume.

Ventilatory changes during laparoscopic cholecystectomy are expected because of the mechanical changes induced by the pneumoperitoneum, changes in the distribution of ventilation and perfusion that result from positioning changes, and systemic absorption of carbon dioxide gas used for insufflation. During pneumoperitoneum, intrathoracic, peak and plateau airway pressure increase in response to an intra-abdominal pressure elevation of 15 mmHg. In patients with normal respiratory function, an increase in peak airway pressure of 15 cmH$_2$O to 23 cmH$_2$O is of little physiologic significance.[11] Other studies have measured the changes in respiratory gas exchange during laparoscopy (Table 7-2). In general, under conditions of controlled positive-pressure ventilation, the changes in oxygenation (PaO$_2$, alveolar-arterial oxygen gradient) are small and clinically insignificant. Several studies have demonstrated increased elimination of carbon dioxide,

Table 7-2. Ventilatory Parameters During Laparoscopic Cholecystectomy

	Before Carbon Dixoide Insufflation	During Carbon Dixoide Insufflation
End-tidal CO_2, mmHg	29.3 ± 6.0	34.7 ± 8.8
pH	7.45 ± 0.09	7.33 ± 0.06
$PaCO_2$, mmHg	31.9 ± 8.4	46.0 ± 9.2
PaO_2, mmHg	409.3 ± 121.6	348.8 ± 130.2
PaO_2-PaO_2 gradient, mmHg	263.9 ± 112.0	190 ± 126
Minute ventilation, ml/kg/min	83.2 ± 18.2	100.0 ± 21.9
Peak inspiratory pressure, cmH_2O	16.0 ± 1.4	25.7 ± 5.5

Abbreviations: $PaCO_2$, partial pressure of carbon dioxide in arterial blood; PaO_2, partial pressure of oxygen in alveolar gas; PaO_2, partial pressure of oxygen in arterial blood. Values are means ± SD.
(Data from Wittgen et al.[10])

reflecting systemic absorption of the carbon dioxide gas used for the pneumoperitoneum. Arterial carbon dioxide tension increases during this time, which may not correlate closely with end-tidal measurement of carbon dioxide. One study concluded that a 15 percent increase in minute ventilation was required to maintain a constant level of carbon dioxide tension during the laparoscopic procedure.[12]

In patients with reactive or obstructive lung disease, the changes in oxygenation and ventilation may be greater than in patients with normal pulmonary function.[10] With lung disease, maldistribution of effective ventilation may increase during the pneumoperitoneum and Trendelenburg position, which may impair oxygenation and/or carbon dioxide elimination. Noninvasive monitoring with pulse oximetry and end-tidal carbon dioxide measurement is sufficient in patients with normal lung function. In patients with pulmonary disease, arterial cannulation will allow repeated blood gas measurements during the operative and postoperative period in order to assess gas exchange.

Oxygenation and ventilation must be monitored closely during the pneumoperitoneum. Pulse oximetry allows noninvasive assessment of oxygenation; end-tidal carbon dioxide measurement via capnography allows an estimate of adequacy of ventilation. In addition, changes in measured expired minute ventilation and peak inspiratory pressure should be noted. Patients with pulmonary disease (identified from symptoms, smoking history, physical examination, or chest radiograph) are more likely to exhibit abnormal gas exchange and ventilation. Additional monitoring (e.g., arterial catheter for measurement of arterial blood gas) may be warranted. Attention should be directed at the best method to increase minute ventilation without adversely changing peak inspiratory pressure and/or intrathoracic pressure. Heightened vigilance is required to detect inadequate ventilation or barotrauma resulting from the pneumoperitoneum.

The anesthesia team must be prepared to manage the rare serious complication. Intra-abdominal hemorrhage may result in cardiovascular collapse at a point where diagnosis and control of hemorrhage may be difficult. Adequate intravenous access (18- or 16-gauge peripheral intravenous line) and close hemodynamic monitoring are indicated. Any abrupt changes in vital signs should be immediately communicated to the surgical team.

A variety of problems require conversion to an open procedure. The anesthesia team should be prepared to handle any changes associated with rapid decompression of the pneumoperitoneum and a laparotomy incision. Attention to vital signs, changes in ventilation, and anesthetic depth is required. During the conversion, hypotension may develop from acutely decreased SVR as the pneumoperitoneum is decompressed or from hypovolemia resulting from bleeding. Acute hypertension and tachycardia may develop if the depth of anesthesia is inadequate for the increased surgical stimulation associated with the open procedure. If hemorrhage is substantial, fluid resuscitation must be rapid, and the blood bank should be notified to cross-match blood.

Intraoperative Monitoring

Routine monitoring for patients undergoing laparoscopic surgery includes noninvasive automated blood pressure, ECG, pulse oximetry, precordial and/or esophageal stethoscope, inspired oxygen concentration, and esophageal temperature. Respiratory gas monitoring, when available, provides valuable information, including end-tidal carbon dioxide and anesthetic agent concentrations. Measurement of end-tidal gas concentrations allows the anesthetist to judge the adequacy of ventilation and the relative depth of anes-

Table 7-3. Anesthetic Plan for Laparoscopic Procedures

Preoperative Assessment and Preparation
Patient evaluation
    History
    Physical examination
    Appropriate diagnostic studies
Assessment
    Cardiopulmonary function, risk of aspiration of gastric contents
Type and screen sample to blood bank

Anesthetic Management
Anesthesia machine, equipment, medications checked
Verify: NPO status, consent
Establish peripheral IV access, invasive monitoring if indicated
Aspiration prophylaxis if indicated
    Antacids, H_2-antagonists, propulsive agents
Premedication (anxiolytics, opioids)
Routine monitoring
    ECG, NIBP, S_pO_2, stethoscope
    Temperature, FiO_2, nerve stimulator
    End-tidal gas monitoring
Preoxygenation, induction of anesthesia
Endotracheal intubation
    Confirmation with breath sounds and capnography
Anesthetic maintenance (inhalation and/or intravenous agents)
Muscle relaxation titrated to peripheral nerve stimulator
Consider antiemetic prophylaxis
Anticipate
    Hemodynamic changes, surgical stimulation
    Trocar insertion, position changes, pneumoperitoneum
Monitor adequacy of ventilation: adjustments as required
Analgesic administration
    Small amounts of opioids
    Consider nonsteroidal anti-inflammatory agents
Vigilance
    Acute intraoperative complications (barotrauma, hemorrhage)

(Continues)

Table 7-3. *(Continued)*

Postoperative Care

Appropriate monitoring during postanesthetic period
    Recovery unit (majority of patients) *or*
    Intensive care (patients with invasive monitoring, etc.)
Assess and treat postoperative nausea and vomiting if present
Appropriate administration
    Intravenous fluids
    Analgesics
    Supplemental oxygen
Assess patient for discharge requirements
    Short stay hospitalization (8–16 hours) *or*
    Consider discharge to home

Abbreviations: ECG, electrocardiogram; FIO$_2$, fraction of inspired oxygen; IV, intravenous; NIBP, automated noninvase blood pressure; S$_p$O$_2$, arterial oxygen saturation by pulse oximetry.

thesia. A peripheral nerve stimulator provides a way to gauge the effects of paralytic agents so doses can be adjusted.

Additional monitors are used as warranted by the patient's medical condition or the type of surgical procedure. Direct intra-arterial measurement of arterial pressure provides beat-to-beat systemic arterial pressures, and the line allows for serial measurement of arterial blood gases. An arterial line is also useful in patients with cardiopulmonary disease or sepsis in whom the induction of anesthesia, position changes, or creation of pneumoperitoneum may give exaggerated hemodynamic responses.

Measurement of central venous pressure, pulmonary artery pressure, pulmonary capillary wedge pressure, and cardiac output can provide valuable information in patients with severe hemodynamic derangements. The additional information regarding intravascular and intraventricular volume status provided by a pulmonary artery catheter may be useful to gauge the response to surgery, anesthesia, and drug therapy. Because patients this ill will most often be cared for in the intensive care unit, they probably will need indwelling Foley catheters to monitor their urine output.

New forms of intraoperative monitoring include transesophageal echocardiography and noninvasive assessment of cardiac output (thoracic bioimpedance, thoracic ultrasound), but the value of these devices during laparoscopic surgery has not been demonstrated. They allow rapid assessment of cardiac status without central intravascular catheters.

Anesthetic Techniques

A standard anesthetic plan is outlined in Table 7-3. General anesthesia and controlled ventilation provide the most stable and flexible approach. Before the patient enters the operating room, a peripheral intravenous cannula is placed, and premedication is administered (e.g., midazolam, 0.5 to 2.0 mg intravenously) to provide anxiolysis and mild sedation. The patient is transferred to the operating table, positioned, and secured with a safety strap. Blood pressure cuff, ECG electrodes, pulse oximeter, and precordial stethoscope are applied, and baseline measurements are obtained before the induction of anesthesia. The patient is allowed to breathe 100 percent oxygen for 2 to 3 minutes to denitrogenate the lungs. Of the many induction agents available, a short-acting sedative hypnotic agent (thiopental, methohexital, propofol) is most often selected. This is often supplemented with a small amount of an opioid (e.g., fentanyl 1 to 3 µg/kg) to blunt the hemodynamic stimulation associated with laryngoscopy and intubation. Patients who could have a full stomach (emergency procedures, active peptic ulcer disease, delayed gastric emptying, symptomatic gastroesophageal reflux) usually undergo a rapid induction of anesthesia in which cricoid pressure is applied as the induction dose of anesthetic is given. The cricoid pressure should be continued until the airway is secured with an endotracheal tube. The latter may be facilitated by a paralytic agent. Following induction and endotracheal intubation, a urinary catheter may be inserted to decompress the bladder, improve abdominal exposure, and monitor urine output. An esophageal stethoscope is used to monitor heart tones and breath sounds, and it allows core body temperature to be measured at the distal esophagus. An oral or nasogastric tube is placed to keep the stomach collapsed. Prophylactic antibiotics may be given at the preference of the surgeon.

Anesthesia is maintained by giving additional anesthetic agents, such as a gas (nitrous oxide), potent inhalational vapors (isoflurane, enflurane, halothane, desflurane, sevoflurane), intravenous opioids (fentanyl, sufentanil, alfentanil, morphine, meperidine), and a variety of intravenous anesthetics (thiopental, methohexital, propofol, ketamine, etomidate). The selection of the specific agents and combinations of agents typically reflects the preferences of the anesthetist and style of anesthesia thought best for the patient. Some newer anesthetic agents allow a faster recovery. Future studies will undoubtedly suggest certain protocols that appear to have desirable features for laparoscopic procedures.

Whether nitrous oxide should be used in laparoscopic surgery remains controversial.[14] An increase in bowel gas may be observed with this agent, and most surgeons prefer that nitrous oxide be avoided. Furthermore, there is a theoretical risk that nitrous oxide could explode in response to contact with the electrocautery. On the other hand, many patients have undergone surgery while receiving nitrous oxide, and no complications have occurred.[11]

Succinylcholine is a depolarizing muscle relaxant with a rapid onset of action and short duration of effect. Because of these properties, it is commonly selected as the paralytic agent to facilitate intubation. Its side effects include fasciculations, myalgias, dysrhythmias, and hyperkalemia. Succinylcholine results in a higher incidence of neck pain and muscle ache compared with nondepolarizing relaxants.[15] Nondepolarizing muscle relaxants have fewer side effects, but onset of action is slower and duration of effect longer. Of the nondepolarizing relaxants, mivacurium, rocuronium, atracurium, and vecuronium have the best features for laparoscopic surgery. Mivacurium has an onset time of 90 to 120 seconds and a short duration of action. It can be administered by incremental bolus injection or continuous infusion. Because the effects are short-lived, it may not require reversal with anticholinesterase agents, which may decrease postoperative nausea and vomiting. Rocuronium has the most rapid onset of action (60 to 90 seconds), and it may be used as an alternative to succinylcholine when a rapid effect is indicated. Atracurium and vecuronium produce effects within 2 to 4 minutes depending on dose. Because of the rapid closure in laparoscopic surgery, short- or intermediate-acting nondepolarizing agents may be preferred to long-acting agents (pancuronium, curare, pipecuronium, doxacurium). Use of a peripheral nerve stimulator helps titrate the dose of muscle relaxant.

Intravenous fluid requirements are markedly less during laparoscopic general surgical procedures compared with open procedures. The standard administration rate of 10 ml/kg/h during open procedures, would be excessive during closed laparoscopic procedures, where 4 to 6 ml/kg/h is sufficient. Obviously, additional fluid may be required if the patient comes to the operating room depleted or becomes hypovolemic.

Thoracoscopic Procedures

Thoracoscopic procedures have many similarities to open thoracic procedures from the anesthetic perspective. Most importantly, to provide adequate exposure, one-lung ventilation is required. Some surgeons still insufflate carbon dioxide to compress the lung, but that is unnecessary and the practice is declining. The anesthesiologist must manage the airway, ventilation, and hemodynamics.[4,5] One-lung ventilation can be done with a double-lumen endotracheal tube, intentional bronchial main stem intubation, or bronchial blockers. Placement of these devices is best confirmed by fiber-optic bronchoscopy. During one-lung ventilation, problems with oxygenation and carbon dioxide elimination are relatively common, particularly in patients with underlying pulmonary disease. Use of high inspired oxygen concentrations, positive end-expiratory pressure in the ventilated lung, or continuous positive airway pressure in the nonventilated lung may be required for adequate oxygenation. Continuous monitoring with pulse oximetry is essential. The ventilatory and carbon dioxide status may be followed with end-tidal gas measurements, but it is best confirmed with direct arterial blood gas measurements. Hemodynamic changes, including hypotension and ectopy, are common during procedures that involve cardiac or mediastinal compression or carbon dioxide insufflation. An arterial cannula for direct measurement of arterial pressure and measurement of arterial blood gases is indicated during most thoracoscopic procedures.

Postoperative Analgesia

Pain is common following most operations, but it is much less following laparoscopic procedures. The anesthetist should administer enough analgesic agents in the operating room and the postanesthesia recovery unit to provide for pain relief. Although opioids, particularly morphine and meperidine, are used most commonly, nonsteroidal anti-inflammatory agents (ketorolac, naproxen, ibuprofen) may be sufficient.[16] Parenteral analgesics are rarely necessary after the patient leaves the recovery room.

Local anesthetics may be used to supplement analgesics. Specifically, consideration should be given to infiltrating local anesthetics (e.g., 0.25 to 0.5 percent bupivacaine) at port sites to reduce incisional pain. One study found no benefit from intraperitoneal local anesthetic administered at the end of a laparoscopic procedure compared with a saline control group. Epidural analgesia and intercostal nerve blocks, effective modalities in providing postoperative analgesia following open cholecystectomy, are not necessary following laparoscopic or thoracoscopic operations.

Postanesthesia Care

Following emergence from the anesthetic, the patient is transported via gurney to the postanesthesia care unit (PACU). Here, care is transferred from the anesthetist to the postanesthesia nurse. During this recovery period, the patient is expected to return to normal consciousness and awareness, which may require 30 to 90 minutes depending on the anesthetic agents, duration of operation, age of the patient, and co-existing illness. Residual anesthetics may impair protective mechanisms against hypoxia and may produce respiratory depression. Upper airway obstruction may develop in the PACU from effects of residual anesthetic and or muscle relaxant. Consequently, supplemental oxygen is usually administered through nasal cannula, oxygen saturation is monitored, and the nurse checks for airway patency. The patient may require additional analgesics, which usually consists of intravenous morphine or meperidine. As many as half of patients may experience nausea, which occasionally requires treatment with droperidol, prochlormethazine, or ondansetron (a $5\text{-}HT_3$ antagonist).

The patient may be discharged from the recovery area when consciousness and vital signs are normal. After laparoscopic cholecystectomy, the patient usually remains hospitalized overnight, but same-day discharge is popular is some areas. The difference is more a matter of concern for immediate abdominal complications than recovery from the anesthetic. A regular diet can be started the same day as surgery as soon as the patient wishes to eat.

References

1. Rose DK, Cohen MM, Soutter DI: Laparoscopic cholecystectomy: the anaesthetist's point of view. Can J Anaesth 39:809, 1992
2. Cunningham AJ, Brull SJ: Laparoscopic cholecystectomy: anesthetic implications. Anesth Analg 76:1120, 1993

3. Hanley ES: Anesthesia for laparoscopic surgery. Surg Clin North Am 72:1013, 1992

4. Lamb JD: Anaesthesia for thoracoscopic pulmonary lobectomy. Can J Anaesth 40:1073, 1993

5. Millar FA, Hutchison GL, Wood RA: Anaesthesia for thoracoscopic pleurectomy and ligation of bullae. Anaesthesia 47:1060, 1992

6. Brown DR, Fishburne JI, Roberson VO, Hulka JF: Ventilatory and blood gas changes during laparoscopy with local anethesia, Am J Obstet Gynecol 124:741, 1977

7. Goodwin AP, Rowe WL, Ogg TW: Day case laparoscopy. A comparison of two anaesthetic techniques using the laryngeal mask during spontaneous breathing. Anaesthesia 47:892, 1992

8. Brimacombe J, Shorney N. Laparoscopy and the laryngeal mask airway? Anaesth Intensive Care 20:245, 1992

9. Safran D, Sgambati S, Orlando R3. Laparoscopy in high-risk cardiac patients. Surg Gynecol Obstet 176:548, 1993

10. Wittgen CM, Andrus CH, Fitzgerald SD et al: Analysis of the hemodynamic and ventilatory effects of laparoscopic cholecystectomy. Arch Surg 126:997, 1991

11. Joris JL, Noirot DP, Legrand MJ et al: Hemodynamic changes during laparoscopic cholecystectomy. Anesth Analg 76:1067, 1993

12. Wahba RW, Mamazza J: Ventilatory requirements during laparoscopic cholecystectomy. Can J Anaesth 40:206, 1993

13. Cunningham AJ, Turner J, Rosenbaum S, Rafferty T: Transoesophageal echocardiographic assessment of haemodynamic function during laparoscopic cholecystectomy. Br J Anaesth 70:621, 1993

14. Thomas DV: Nitrous oxide should not be used during laparoscopy nor during other abdominal operations, letter, comment. Anaesthesia 47:80, 1992.

15. Smith I, Ding Y, White PF: Muscle pain after outpatient laparoscopy—influence of propofol versus thiopental and enflurane. Anesth Analg 76:1181, 1993

16. Liu J, Ding Y, White PF et al: Effects of ketorolac on postoperative analgesia and ventilatory function after laparoscopic cholecystectomy. Anesth Analg 76:1061, 1993

8

▶ Complications

S. H. Carvajal
S. J. Mulvihill
L. W. Way

IMPROVEMENTS IN VIDEO AND LAPAROSCOPIC INSTRUMENTATION HAVE made it possible to perform many abdominal operations laparoscopically. The driving force for adoption of laparoscopic operations has been their benefits in regard to postoperative pain, length of hospital stay, and time off work.[1,2] Indeed, the laparoscopic approach has replaced open surgery as the procedure of choice for elective cholecystectomy.

The benefits must be weighed against the complications resulting from the new laparoscopic techniques and instruments. The risk-to-benefit ratio must be analyzed for each laparoscopic operation, and the risks must be compared with those of the alternative open operations. Complicating this analysis is the reality that the risks are greater early in a surgeon's experience with a new laparoscopic operation.[1–3]

The most worrisome technical complications of laparoscopic surgery stem from many factors, including (1) two-dimensional video imaging, (2) an unfamiliar operative view that differs from open surgery, and (3) limited instrumental motion and feedback.[4]

Complications may be categorized as those unique to laparoscopic surgery and those that also occur during open surgery. The former may be subdivided into those related to the pneumoperitoneum, patient position, or instrumentation (Table 8-1).

Table 8-1. Summary of Laparoscopic Complications

Classification	Complication
Complications unique to laparoscopy	
Related to pneumoperitoneum	Hypercarbia, acidosis
	Ventilation/perfusion mismatching
	Hypertension
	Bradyarrhythmias
	Ventricular arrhythmias
	Gas embolism
	Pneumothorax
	Pneumomediastinum
	Subcutaneous emphysema
	Phlebothrombosis and pulmonary embolism
Related to position	Neuropathy
	Hypotension
Related to instrumentation	Trocar and Veress needle injuries of the intestine or major blood vessels
	Abdominal wall bleeding
	Trocar site hernia
	Electrocautery or laser burns
	Wound infections
	Retractor injury
Complications of specific operations	
Laparoscopic cholecystectomy	Bile duct injury
	Bile fistula
	Hemorrhage
	Intraperitoneal gallstones
	Retained common duct stones
Laparoscopic appendectomy	Abdominal abscess
	Wound infection
	Appendiceal rupture
Laparoscopic colectomy	Trocar site recurrence
	Bowel injury
	Ureteral injury
	Duodenal injury
Laparoscopic herniorrhaphy	Recurrence
	Bowel erosion
	Mesh infection
	Nerve entrapment
Laparoscopic antireflux procedures	Perforated esophagus
	Vagus nerve injury
	Pneumothorax
	Dysphagia
	Gas bloat
	Paraesophageal hernia

Complications Related to Pneumoperitoneum

The exposure required to perform laparoscopic surgery chiefly depends on establishing an adequate pneumoperitoneum. The insufflated gas separates the abdominal wall from the underlying viscera, and the laparoscope and laparoscopic instruments are inserted into the resulting space. Although it may cause respiratory and cardiovascular physiologic changes, the pneumoperitoneum produces no adverse effects in most patients.

Carbon dioxide is the gas most often used to create the pneumoperitoneum. Compared with ordinary air, carbon dioxide does not support combustion, which permits electrocautery and lasers to be used, and carbon dioxide readily diffuses into blood, which minimizes the risk of gas embolism.[5]

Metabolic Effects of Carbon Dioxide (See Also Ch. 7)

Peritoneal absorption of carbon dioxide may produce hypercarbia and acidosis, which have been reported to cause ventricular arrhythmias in as many as 17 percent of patients undergoing laparoscopy.[6,7] Hypercarbia may also stimulate sympathetic discharge, which increases systemic vascular resistance, contractility, and mean arterial pressure.[8] Acidosis has been associated with other sequelae, including precipitation of sickle cell crisis in patients with sickle cell disease. In healthy patients, mild acidosis is well tolerated, and hypercapnia can be corrected by increasing the minute ventilation. In patients with chronic lung disease or cardiovascular disease, however, hypercarbia and acidosis may continue despite correction of hypercapnia.[9,10] Acidosis may be pronounced in hypovolemic patients (e.g., during diagnostic laparoscopy for trauma[11]). For patients in whom acidosis would be a risk, arterial pH and $PaCO_2$ should be monitored frequently during the pneumoperitoneum, and appropriate ventilatory changes should be made to correct hypercarbia and acidosis.

Pulmonary Effects

Cephalad displacement of the diaphragm by the pneumoperitoneum may decrease functional residual capacity and total lung capacity.[12] The resulting atelectasis of the lung bases may cause ventilation-perfusion mismatching, further contributing to hypoventilation. These changes lead to an elevated mean airway pressure and diminished pulmonary compliance.[13] Diaphragmatic displacement and the resulting physiologic changes are greatest when the patient is in steep Trendelenburg position, which is used, for example, in laparoscopic pelvic operations. Mechanical ventilation effectively counteracts these pulmonary effects in most cases, and keeping intra-abdominal pressure within the recommended range (less than 15 mmHg) also helps.

After the pneumoperitoneum has been decompressed, hypercarbia may persist for up to 3 hours as a result of continued diaphragmatic dysfunction or reabsorption of residual carbon dioxide.[14] Because it may occur with open as well as laparoscopic cholecystectomy, diaphragmatic dysfunction cannot be entirely attributed to the pneumoperitoneum.[15] To prevent reabsorption hypercarbia, the pneumoperitoneum should be thoroughly evacuated at the end of the case, and the patient should be monitored for signs of hypercarbia.

Pneumothorax and pneumomediastinum may develop as a result of injury to the diaphragm, mediastinal pleura (e.g., during esophageal dissection), or anatomic defects in the diaphragm or esophageal hiatus. In addition, under the increased pressure, gas may dissect through the retroperitoneal tissues into the mediastinum or pleura.[16] Pneumomediastinum rarely affects hemodynamics. On the other hand, tension pneumothorax may increase mean airway pressure, desaturate arterial blood, and produce cardiac collapse.[17] Treatment consists of a thoracostomy tube. In the absence of physiologic sequelae, however, a carbon dioxide pneumothorax may be managed expectantly as carbon dioxide readily diffuses through the pleura.[18]

Hemodynamic Effects

Intra-abdominal pressures above 20 mmHg can increase central venous pressure, decrease central venous return, and diminish cardiac output.[19,20] Systemic vascular resistance may also rise as a result of mechanical compression of the splanchnic capillary beds.[21] In contrast, minor elevations of intra-abdominal pressure may increase venous return by compressing the viscera and vena cava.[20]

Bradycardia, the most common arrhythmia (in 30 percent of cases) is thought to be caused by abdominal wall distension and peritoneal irritation leading to vagal discharge.[22] Other possible bradyarrhythmias include atrioventricular dissociation, nodal rhythms, and asystole.

All of these hemodynamic changes may be exacerbated by the extreme positions often needed during laparoscopic surgery. To avoid serious complications, patients with limited cardiac reserve should be monitored with arterial and possibly pulmonary artery catheters.

Extraperitoneal Insufflation

Insufflating through a Veress needle whose tip is in the abdominal wall may lead to subcutaneous emphysema, which can occasionally be massive. While usually of no serious consequence, it rarely results in pneumothorax, pneumomediastinum, or hypercarbia.[23,24] The most common site of incorrect insufflation is the preperitoneal space, an error that is usually diagnosed when the laparoscope is placed into the preperitoneal space. To remedy the problem, the preperitoneal gas should be removed (to the extent possible) and a pneumoperitoneum created using an open (Hasson) technique. Bowel penetration with the Veress needle may result in insufflation of bowel and asymmetric abdominal distension. If as a result the bowel becomes greatly distended, the laparoscopic approach may have to be abandoned.

Gas Embolism

Despite carbon dioxide's high diffusion coefficient, hypotension may result from carbon dioxide embolism.[25,26] The usual cause of gas embolism is insufflation through a Veress needle inserted into a major vessel. Some cases are postulated to have resulted from carbon dioxide diffusing through dissected tissue and collecting in the right atrium where it produced a gas lock.[27] A substantial amount of carbon dioxide must enter the veins, however, for gas embolism to occur. For example, as much as 0.1 L/min has been reported to have no serious physiologic effects.[28] Carbon dioxide embolism causes acute hypotension and a mill wheel murmur. Treatment consists of immediate deflation of the pneumoperitoneum and placing the patient in a steep left lateral decubitus Trendelenburg position. A venous catheter should then be threaded into the right atrium and the gas evacuated. If gas lock continues, median sternotomy and drainage of the gas in the pulmonary outflow may be necessary. Cardiopulmonary bypass has been used successfully for carbon dioxide embolism.[25] Other causes of acute cardiovascular collapse should be ruled out, including hemorrhage, pneumothorax, myocardial infarction, vagal discharge, arrhythmia, and anaphylaxis (see below).

Deep Venous Thrombosis

Deep venous thrombosis is a theoretical risk. In one study, induction of a pneumoperitoneum regularly decreased common femoral venous flow, an

Causes of Sudden Cardiovascular Collapse During Laparoscopic Surgery

Trocar injury to major vessel and hemorrhage

Gas embolism

Tension pneumothorax

Asystole secondary to vagal stimulation from abdominal distension

Ventricular arrhythmia secondary to hypercarbia and acidosis

Excessive pneumoperitoneum pressure

Myocardial infarction

Anaphylaxis

effect that could be reversed by intermittent sequential pneumatic compression of the lower extremities.[29] In general, however, the risk of deep venous thrombosis and pulmonary embolism appears to be no higher following laparoscopy than laparotomy.[30] The diagnosis of pulmonary embolism may be difficult, because the presenting signs may be overlooked or dismissed as a result of right upper quadrant surgery. Preventive measures such as preoperative breathing exercises, subcutaneous heparin, and intraoperative graduated compression stockings should be considered as in open surgery.

Alternative Gases

Nitrous oxide and helium have been suggested as alternative gases for the pneumoperitoneum.[31] Neither has the potential of hypercarbia and acidosis.[32] Nitrous oxide has the theoretical risk of supporting combustion, but no intra-abdominal explosions have been reported. Helium is inert and incapable of supporting combustion. Diffusion of both helium and nitrous oxide in blood is poor compared with carbon dioxide, so theoretically, both have a higher risk of gas embolism. Nitrous oxide is an anesthetic, and its use may reduce other anesthetic requirements.[33] Despite these points, there is presently no enthusiasm for shifting to either of these alternatives.

Alternatives to the Pneumoperitoneum

Abdominal wall lifting devices are available, and their use is discussed in Chapter 2. Exposure remains compromised enough with the current mechanical lift systems that the risk of technical complications is increased and operations are more difficult.

Complications Related to Position

Pelvic operations may require a steep Trendelenburg position to displace the omentum and intestines from the pelvis. To prevent the patient from sliding off the table, shoulder braces are commonly used with the patient's arms abducted. Because brachial plexus injuries have been reported,[34–36] we recommend placing the patient on a beanbag mattress secured to the operative table. This prevents the patient from slipping without using braces.

Femoral nerve mononeuropathies have been reported in patients placed in the lithotomy position.[37] The lesions were localized to the inguinal ligament and probably occurred as a result of nerve compression by the ligament. In other cases, the femoral nerve may have been stretched by excessive hip abduction and external rotation. Peroneal neuropathy is another rare complication. Nerve injury during lithotomy position may be prevented by careful positioning and padding of the lower extremities and avoiding excessive hip abduction and external rotation. The hemodynamic changes related to patient position are summarized in Table 7-1.

Complications Related to Instrumentation

In the usual closed method of laparoscopic access (see Ch. 3), the Veress needle and first trocar are inserted blindly. Although the recommended technique incorporates steps intended to avoid complications, underlying viscera or blood vessels may rarely be penetrated. Although the use of disposable Veress needles and trocars with protective, spring-loaded, blunt covers (safety shields) may decrease the incidence of these injuries,[8] serious and occasionally fatal injuries have been reported despite the use of trocars with safety shields. The reported incidence of visceral injures is 0.025 to 0.2 percent.[38–41] In general, penetration of a viscus by the Veress needle is well tolerated. The needle is simply backed out. On the other hand, penetration of a retroperitoneal blood vessel by the Veress needle, or any visceral or retroperitoneal blood vessel by the trocar, is potentially life threatening unless detected promptly and repaired.[42]

Vascular Injury

The bifurcation of the aorta lies beneath the umbilicus, and it and the iliac vessels are vulnerable. The vena cava is less likely to be injured because of its posterolateral location in reference to the aorta. In children and thin adults, these vessels may lie only 2 to 3 cm below the abdominal wall. The reported incidence of vascular injury that is due to needle or trocar insertion is 0.017 to 0.05 percent,[39–41] and the mortality rate is 8.8 to 13 percent.[40,43] The principal causes of injury to major vessels are overshoot when inserting the umbilical trocar, incomplete pneumoperitoneum (so the abdominal wall is not taut), incomplete relaxation (so the abdominal wall is too close to the vessels), and failure to insert the trocar at a 45° angle (so the path between the abdominal wall and vessels is short).

Veress needle entry into a major vessel is often diagnosed by aspiration with a syringe. Although the puncture may be small and the bleeding minor and self-contained, the risks of assuming so are enormous. It is more difficult than imagined to assess the size and stability of a retroperitoneal hematoma laparoscopically. A presumed puncture of the vena cava may actually be a laceration. Punctures of the aorta or iliac arteries may not seal spontaneously, especially in the elderly. Consequently, we recommend that the abdomen be opened and the retroperitoneum carefully inspected and observed if there is any evidence that the Veress needle has entered a major vessel. Injuries that are actively bleeding should be exposed and repaired. Delay in diagnosis of retroperitoneal bleeding markedly increases the risk of death.

Major vessel injury from the trocar most often presents with visible hemorrhage or unexplained hypotension.[43] If this complication is suspected, a laparotomy should be performed immediately. Because the hole is so large, trocar injuries to the aorta may be fatal, even if promptly recognized and treated. In most cases, however, the bleeding is contained in the retroperitoneum for a time before it erupts into the abdominal cavity, which provides an opportunity to get it under control if the diagnosis is made. Failure to consider the diagnosis soon enough and to look for corroborating evidence has been an element in most fatal cases. Repair of the injury may require placement of an allograft or, in serious venous injury, may require ligation of the inferior vena cava below the renal veins.

Bowel Injury

The reported incidence of bowel injury is 0.06 to 0.14 percent,[39,40] and the mortality rate is about 5 percent.[42] Veress needle injuries may occur fairly often, but because they produce no complications and do not require repair, they may go unrecognized or unreported.[33,44] Trocar injuries require immediate open repair. Diagnosis is usually made when bowel contents escape from the trocar or when the lumen is seen after the laparoscope is inserted. The trocar should be left in place while the abdomen is opened, because it may otherwise be difficult to find the perforation simply by running the intestine from top to bottom. Furthermore, two or more injuries may be caused by skewering adjacent loops of bowel. One or more of these enterotomies could be overlooked as more obvious ones are discovered. This is also why laparoscopic repair is not usually appropriate.

Disposable needles and trocars are designed to limit the risk of bowel injury, but their efficacy in this respect is unproved. The technique of needle and trocar insertion is very important (see Ch. 3). Major risk factors for bowel perforation are previous abdominal operation, history of peritonitis, bowel distension, and presence of metastatic disease.[16,40] When these risk factors are present, it is safest to use the open (Hasson) laparoscopic technique. The risk of stomach perforation can be minimized by decompressing the stomach with a nasogastric tube before needle insertion.

Bladder Injury

Bladder injury from a Veress needle or trocar is rare.[5] Decompressing the bladder with a Foley catheter helps with prevention. The risk is increased by previous bladder surgery, congenital anomalies, or previous low abdominal operation. Manifestations include aspiration of urine, pneumaturia, or hematuria.[45] A trocar injury should be repaired.

Solid Organ and Mesenteric Injury

Injuries may occur to the spleen, liver, and mesentery. Carbon dioxide insufflation in these organs may cause cardiac collapse secondary to gas embolism.

The open Hasson technique may be appropriate in some patients with an enlarged spleen or liver.

Abdominal Wall Bleeding

Bleeding can result from injury to an abdominal wall vessel by a trocar. This usually occurs during placement of accessory trocars and can be recognized by noting blood dripping from the trocar into the operative field or bleeding from the wound in the abdominal wall as the trocar is removed. These injuries may be avoided by identifying the epigastric vessels (with the laparoscope) by transilluminating the abdominal wall and placing the trocars to miss them.[44] The presence of periumbilical varices (caput medusa) makes patients with portal hypertension at high risk of bleeding during trocar insertion, so the Hasson technique might be preferred.

Most trocar site bleeding stops spontaneously, but if it does not, hemostasis may be obtained by tamponade with a Foley catheter balloon or with sutures. The Foley method involves removing the trocar, inserting the catheter through the tract, and inflating the (50-cc) balloon within the abdomen. Traction is exerted on the catheter so the balloon compresses the bleeder. It may take 30 minutes or more before the traction can be released without having the bleeding resume. The suture technique is described in Chapter 3. If these methods are unsuccessful, the skin incision may be enlarged so the vessel can be ligated.[33]

Trocar Site Herniation

Trocar site hernias may trap omentum or bowel,[46–50] often as a Richter's hernia. Hernias are rare through 5-mm port sites and uncommon through 10-mm port sites, but they occur in about 2 percent of 12-mm port sites, especially in the lower abdomen. The presentation consists of pain and small bowel obstruction 3 to 5 days postoperatively. This complication can be prevented by adequate closure of the large trocar wounds, but an adequate closure in the lower abdomen must include all layers of the abdominal wall, not just the most superficial layer of fascia. (The technique is described in Ch. 3.) Furthermore, trocars should be withdrawn under direct vision with the laparoscope to ensure that bowel or omentum is not pulled into the wound. It has been postulated that inserting the trocars using a zigzag technique might decrease the risk of herniation,[8] but this method is less feasible with the larger trocars, which in turn are most susceptible to hernia formation.

Injury Resulting From Electrocautery and Lasers

Electrocautery and lasers may accidentally produce injuries of the blood vessels and viscera.[40,51,52] Contact injuries may result in perforation of the bowel or stricture formation in the bile duct.[54,55] Typically, injuries to vessels cause immediate hemorrhage, but they may also lead to late pseudoaneurysm formation.[55] Complication rates with laser and monopolar electrocautery are no different.[2,40,56,57] Many of these injuries may be prevented just by using the devices correctly. The classification of these injuries, their mechanism, and the appropriate use of these instruments are discussed in Chapters 2 and 3.

Wound Infections

Wound infections are rare in laparoscopic surgery, probably because the incisions are so small. Studies have shown that carbon dioxide does not inhibit bacterial growth, as was once proposed.[58] Wound abscesses do occur occasionally, and necrotizing fasciitis following diagnostic laparotomy has also been reported.[59] The risk of wound infection can be minimized by placing infected tissue (e.g., the appendix) in extraction bags. Avoiding abdominal wall hematomas through good hemostasis also helps.

Retractor and Grasper Injury

During advanced laparoscopic procedures, retractors are needed to displace organs such as liver, spleen, and bowel. Injury may occur if force is excessive. Graspers (e.g., Babcock clamps) have been developed to retract bowel, but because tactile feedback is diminished, the forces delivered to the bowel wall may be enough to cause a tear. Torquing injuries, the most common, can be prevented by understanding how they occur and avoiding those circumstances. The design features and use of these instruments should be reviewed (Chs. 2 and 3).

Complications of Mechanical Clips

Dislodgment or inappropriate placement of metal clips has led to bile leaks, hemorrhage, and bile duct injury.[16] Clips can be dislodged easily if distracted or as a result of dissection adjacent to a clip.[60] Clips should be applied precisely, and all clips should be inspected following completion of the operation.

Complications of Specific Procedures

Laparoscopic Cholecystectomy

Bile Duct Injury

Bile duct injury is the most common serious complication of laparoscopic cholecystectomy, occurring in about 0.2 percent of cases.[1,2,40,61,62] The problem may actually be underreported, however.[16] This compares with a bile duct injury of 0.1 percent in open cholecystectomy.[1,3,62,63] Bile duct injury is more likely early in a surgeon's laparoscopic experience.[1-3] In one study, during a surgeon's first 13 laparoscopic cholecystectomies, the risk of bile duct injury was 2.2 percent but declined to 0.1 percent thereafter.[1] The number of patients with bile duct injuries being referred to tertiary care centers appears to be declining,[64] which suggests that the injury rate is dropping (Fig. 8-1).

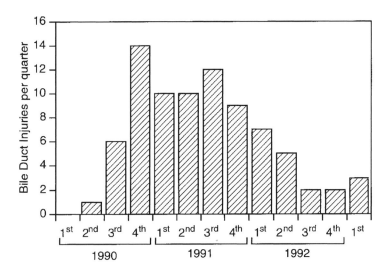

Fig. 8-1. Referrals of patients with bile duct injuries over time to three tertiary care centers. The rate rose rapidly following introduction of laparoscopic cholecystectomy and has subsequently diminished. This suggests that the incidence of laparoscopic cholecystectomy-associated bile duct injuries is decreasing. (Reprinted from Woods et al.,[64] with permission.)

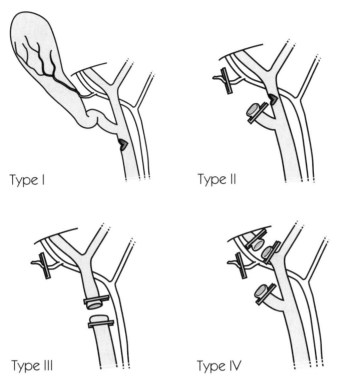

Fig. 8-2. Classification scheme for bile duct injuries (see text).

A classification of bile duct injuries during laparoscopic cholecystectomy has been proposed by Stewart et al.[61] (Fig. 8-2). A type I injury is an incision or incomplete transection of the common bile or common hepatic duct resulting from misidentification of the cystic duct or inadvertent extension of the cystic duct incision. In this injury, the error is diagnosed before complete transection of the duct. A type II injury is a common hepatic duct stricture with or without a fistula, which results from electrocautery injury or clip application on the duct. It usually occurs in attempts to control bleeding from the cystic artery or from imprecise dissection. A type III injury is excision of a central portion of the common duct, including the junction of cystic and common duct. Type IV injuries are confined to the right hepatic duct and consist of occlusion or transection. Type I and III injuries result from misidentification of the common duct as the cystic duct.

Bile duct injury, when diagnosed intraoperatively, should be repaired immediately. Type I injuries should be treated by precise closure with fine (5-0 or 6-0) absorbable sutures, usually without a T-tube. Type II, III, and IV injuries usually require Roux en Y choledochojejunostomy or hepaticojejunostomy. When a bile duct injury is suspected in the postoperative period, an initial ultrasound or CT scan is useful to identify a biloma or occasionally bile duct dilatation. If a collection of fluid is seen, it should be drained percutaneously, which will usually show that it is bile. This serves the dual purpose of diagnosis and control of the bile fistula, which is critical to prevent infection. If a bile leak is suspected, a hepatoiminodiacetic acid (HIDA) scan may also be confirmatory, but this is rarely necessary. Endoscopic retrograde cholangiopancreatography (ERCP) or percutaneous transhepatic cholangiography are necessary to define the lesion and the extrahepatic biliary anatomy. It is reasonable to attempt management of minimal type II injuries by endoscopic or percutaneous biliary dilatation of the stricture, although recurrent stricture formation is common. The outcome of reparative operations for these lesions is much better in tertiary care centers than when performed by the initial surgeon.

Patients may present with clinical manifestations of unrecognized biliary injury from days to months postoperatively, depending on the type and degree of injury. Some patients present with progressive jaundice and only mild biliary pain. Others present with frank cholangitis. About 75 percent of patients with bile duct injury following laparoscopic cholecystectomy present with bile ascites, which causes anorexia, ileus bloating, abdominal distention, and mild hyperbilirubinemia or jaundice. If diagnosed and drained early, the morbidity of bile ascites is usually very little. If diagnosis and drainage is delayed for a few weeks, bile ascites may evolve into bile peritonitis, a much more serious condition.[65] Abdominal computed tomography (CT) or ultrasound typically shows a subphrenic fluid collection or free intraperitoneal fluid, occasionally with dilated bile ducts.

The key to preventing the most common bile duct injuries is to avoid confusing the common duct for the cystic duct. Exposure of Calot's triangle is crucial as the first step in this procedure. This is achieved by *lateral* retraction of the infundibulum of the gallbladder and may be helped by using a 30° laparoscope. Intraoperative cholangiography should be performed routinely in the surgeon's early experience, whenever an anomalous duct is thought to be present, when the anatomy is unclear, and when a chronic inflammation at the base of the gallbladder is considerable, for these are the situations where misidentification of the common duct for the cystic duct is most common.[66–68] Cholangiography also identifies injuries that may have already occurred (class I) and prevents them from being converted to more serious (class III) injuries.

Biliary Fistula Without Common Duct Injury

The most common postoperative complication following laparoscopic chole-cystectomy is biliary leak, with a reported incidence of 0.2 to 1.5 percent.[1,2,40,62] It results from dislodgment of the cystic duct clips, necrosis of the cystic duct stump, or transection of unrecognized ducts of Luschka. Patients may present with pruritus, bile peritonitis, shoulder pain, ileus, abdominal distension, ascites, fever, or jaundice.[2,49,62] Typically, laboratory studies are only remarkable for a mildly elevated direct bilirubin level and leukocytosis. Abdominal CT or ultrasound scans usually demonstrate a subphrenic fluid collection or free intraperitoneal fluid, and aspiration reveals it to be bile. An ERCP should be performed to identify the site of extravasation. Ultrasound or CT-guided percutaneous drainage should be followed by endoscopic place-ment of a temporary stent across the sphincter (which decreases biliary pres-sure). The fistula usually closes within 2 weeks. If a bile leak that is due to clip dislodgment from the cystic duct is identified early in the postoperative period, repeat laparoscopy with aspiration of the bile collection and ligation of the cystic duct stump may be considered. Patients who present late with peritonitis that is due to infected intraperitoneal bile should be treated with laparotomy, irrigation, closure or repair of the fistula, and drainage.

Hemorrhage

The rate of postoperative hemorrhage following laparoscopic cholecystec-tomy ranges from 0.08 to 0.3 percent.[1,2,40] The source may be the liver bed, cystic artery, abdominal wall, or unrecognized major vascular injury. Hemorrhage after the patient has been discharged from the hospital is associ-ated with a high mortality rate. In most instances, major postoperative hemor-rhage requires surgical control by laparotomy. The average blood loss during laparoscopic cholecystectomy is less than 10 ml. If bleeding exceeds 100 to 200 ml, and especially if transfusion is considered, the procedure should often be converted to a laparotomy.

Gallstone Spillage

The gallbladder may rupture during retraction or dissection, and the stones may escape into the abdomen. The rate of gallbladder perforation is approximately 20 percent, and stones are freed in most of these cases.[69] Unretrieved gallstones rarely cause complications, but intra-abdominal abscess formation has been reported.[47] The risk is probably greater with pigment than with cholesterol gallstones. An intraperitoneal gallstone may also erode into an adjacent structure (e.g., bile duct) or even through the abdominal wall via a trocar wound.[8]

Spilled gallstones should be retrieved if possible, but the risks of leaving a stone or two behind are insufficient to justify a laparotomy. A Dormia basket may be used to extract large stones. A bag may be introduced into the abdomen to collect medium-sized stones. Small stones can typically be extracted by suction–irrigation using a large-bore cannula.

Laparoscopic Herniorrhaphy

A survey of 1514 hernia repairs showed the following rates of recurrence after different kinds of repairs: transabdominal preperitoneal hernia repair, 0.7 percent; extra-abdominal preperitoneal repair, 0.4 percent; intra-abdominal onlay mesh, 2.2 percent; and plug/patch repair, 22 percent.[70] An analysis of 60 recurrences in 3353 repairs revealed that 60 percent of recurrences could be attributed to using a mesh too small to cover all potential hernia sites, 32 percent to the mesh not being fixed in place, and 20 percent to a missed hernia. If a large mesh is used and stapled properly, the recurrence rate drops to less than 0.5 percent.[70]

Other reported complications include intraoperative problems (0.1 percent; e.g., hypotension and hemorrhage), local complications (5.3 percent; e.g., hematoma, hydrocele, and infection), nerve entrapment (2.8 percent), urinary tract infection (2.4 percent), and testicular pain and epididymitis (2.3 percent). Currently, laparoscopic hernia repairs require a general anesthetic, whereas the majority of open herniorrhaphies can be performed under local anesthesia, factors that must be considered in the risk analysis. In one series, the only death following laparoscopic herniorrhaphy was due to myocardial infarction.[71]

Most surgeons use staples to fix the mesh to the underlying fascia. Misplaced staples may injure the gonadal, inferior epigastric, and external iliac vessels, the vas deferens, or nearby nerves.[72,73,74] The femoral branch of the genitofemoral nerve and the lateral cutaneous nerve of the thigh appear to be at greatest risk. To avoid injuring these nerves, no staples should be applied wherever counterpressure from the outside cannot deform the site of clip placement (i.e., below the iliopubic tract), except on Cooper's ligament. Entrapment of nerves typically causes severe neuralgia and may require laparoscopic removal of the offending staple. Injury to blood vessels may cause serious hemorrhage that requires a laparotomy for control.

The transabdominal preperitoneal mesh and intraperitoneal onlay mesh repairs both place the patient at risk for intra-abdominal adhesion formation and small bowel obstruction. Because no long-term follow-up is yet available, the incidence of this complication is unknown. In one report of two patients who underwent laparotomy following laparoscopic hernia repair, one patient had numerous omental adhesions to the trocar wounds and only one minor adhesion between a tag of sigmoid omentum and the preperitoneal incision, and the other patient had dense adhesions to the sigmoid colon.[75] The intraperitoneal onlay mesh technique seems most likely to increase the risk of adhesion formation and possibly even erosion of mesh into bowel (although no such instance has been reported). The extraperitoneal approach theoretically has no risk of intra-abdominal adhesion formation. All three repairs use a synthetic polypropylene mesh, which could become infected. Nevertheless, the same kind of mesh has been used in hernia repairs for 30 years, and this complication has been quite rare.

Laparoscopic Appendectomy

The complications of laparoscopic appendectomy include appendiceal rupture, intra-abdominal abscess, prolonged fever, hemorrhage, and appendiceal stump fistula. Wound infection rates following laparoscopic appendectomy average 1 percent.[76–80] In contrast, the incidence of wound infections following open appendectomy is about 6 percent.[78–81] Although most studies report no intra-abdominal abscesses, in two articles, 6 percent of patients developed abscesses following laparoscopic appendectomy.[79,80] Appendiceal rupture during retraction, hemorrhage, and stump leaks were rare.[77,82] The theoretical risks of cecal injury during retraction, bladder injury, or ureteral injury have not been reported.

Laparoscopic Colectomy

Injuries to the ureter, urinary bladder, and duodenum may be more likely in laparoscopic colon surgery because of perspective and technical limitations.[83–85] Among these, ureteral injury is most worrisome because it is especially difficult to identify the ureter laparoscopically. The injury may go unnoticed during the operation. Surgeons have attempted to prevent this complication by deliberately dissecting and identifying the ureter (inducing peristalsis by compressing the ureter with a grasper) early in the dissection, or alternatively by placing stents or even transilluminating the ureter with a ureteroscope placed transurethrally.[86,87] A potential complication of laparoscopic anterior resection is that of anastomotic leak when the anastomosis is created using a circular stapling device. In one report, 18 percent of these mechanical anastomoses needed to be augmented with intracorporeal sutures to prevent anastomotic leakage.[88] This highlights the need to be able to suture before embarking on these advanced laparoscopic procedures.

Several reports have been made of tumor recurring at trocar sites.[89,90] The cause is uncertain but probably relates to extraction of tumor specimens through trocar sites or spillage of tumor cells during laparoscopic dissection. It is of interest that many surgeons who have performed large numbers of laparoscopic colectomies have not encountered this complication, which suggests further that it may be related to technique. The efficacy of laparoscopic surgery for cancer operations cannot be judged until the results of long-term follow-up studies and controlled trials are reported.

Antireflux Procedures

Among the most worrisome complications specific to laparoscopic antireflux procedures are perforation of the esophagus or stomach. Perforations most often occur as a nasogastric tube or bougie is being passed by the anesthesiologist into the stomach, and the device runs into resistance created by an instrument holding the tissue. Babcock clamps and other graspers may also directly perforate the stomach, especially the thin-walled fundus. Instruments to grasp the stomach should have a comparatively large surface area of contact, and the amount of squeeze should be kept to the minimum necessary to hold the tissue. Dissection of the esophagus with pointed instruments is another cause of perforation. Cautery injuries of the stomach have resulted in perforations, which are usually immediate but may not be manifest for 12 to 24 hours postoperatively. The greatest risk is when using monopolar cautery in conjunction with a laparoscopic scissors, because there is a greater length of uninsulated metal on the scissors than on most other instruments.

Vagal nerve injuries stem from misidentification of the nerves, which may then be cut, or from the use of cautery too close to the nerves. In the latter instance, it appears as if the monopolar current uses the nerve as a pathway to ground, and the clinical syndrome consists of delayed gastric emptying (bloating and early satiety) that spontaneously returns to normal within a few months.

Paraesophageal hernia may develop postoperatively with pain, dysphagia, and recurrent reflux as its manifestations. This complication has been seen most commonly when the crural borders have not been approximated to narrow the enlarged hiatus and when technical measures have not been taken to anchor the esophagus and fundoplication wrap within the abdomen.

The proximity of the pleura to the esophagus, especially on the right side, leads to a risk of pneumothorax during the esophageal dissection of an antireflux procedure. The pneumothorax may be noticed by increased airway pressure. Specific treatment, such as placement of a chest tube, is not usually required, because the chest communicates with the abdominal cavity and positive pressure ventilation by the anesthesiologist evacuates most of the gas. Also, the carbon dioxide is absorbed rapidly through the pleura. Placing a chest tube is rarely appropriate, and it may result in enough loss of the pneumoperitoneum that even a high-flow insufflator cannot compensate. On completion of the procedure, the pneumoperitoneum should be evacuated completely while the airway pressure is kept at more than 20 mmHg, which helps evacuate carbon dioxide from the chest and the lung to expand fully. Persistent pneumothorax may be treated by needle aspiration or by placing a chest tube.

A 13 percent complication rate in the immediate postoperative period has been reported for laparoscopic antireflux procedures. Persistent reflux is uncommon. Other symptoms related to the procedure include gas bloat, dysphagia, gastroparesis, and diarrhea.

Postoperative dysphagia and gas bloat may be prevented by taking the following precautions. In particular, it is important to select the most appropriate type of antireflux procedure after taking into consideration the results of preoperative manometric studies (i.e., a partial wrap should be performed for a patient with impaired peristalsis of the esophageal body). The crura should be closed but not too tight around the esophagus (i.e., 1 cm should be left unclosed). Short gastric vessels should be divided, so that the gastric fundus is fully mobilized, which prevents the fundus from being pulled back to its original position, producing lateral traction on the esophagus (and dysphagia). Fixing the wrap to the crura may also offset this force. When creating the wrap, the largest Maloney bougie available (e.g., 50 to 60 French) should be introduced into the esophagus, and the wrap should be short (2 cm) and floppy. Mild dysphagia is still present for a few weeks in many patients, but persistent dysphagia will be rare if these technical principles are adhered to.

Persistent reflux is most often attributed to wrap failure, which includes disrupted, deintussuscepted, and herniated wraps. To prevent the wrap from coming undone, the esophageal muscle should be incorporated into two of the stitches used to create the wrap. Deintussusception of the wrap can be prevented by fixing the cephalad margins of the wrap to the esophagus (i.e., collar stitches). In patients with hiatal hernias, the wrap is at risk of herniating into the chest, which can be prevented by stitches that fix the wrap in the abdomen (i.e., between the wrap and the closed crus; between the sides of the esophagus and the sides of the crural hiatus).

Conclusion

Laparoscopic procedures are associated with complications that can largely be prevented by proper training and by understanding their cause. The incidence of long-term complications will only be known with time.

References

1. The Southern Surgeons Club. A prospective analysis of 1518 laparoscopic cholecystectomies. N Engl J Med 324:1073, 1991
2. Larson GM, Vitale GC, Casey J et al: Multipractice analysis of laparoscopic cholecystectomy in 1,983 patients. Am J Surg 163:221, 1992
3. Davidoff AM, Pappas TN, Murray EA et al: Mechanisms of major biliary injury during laparoscopic cholecystectomy [see comments]. Ann Surg 215:196, 1992
4. Soper NJ, Brunt LM, Kerbl K: Laparoscopic general surgery. N Engl J Med 330:409, 1994

5. Capelouto CC, Kavoussi LR: Complications of laparoscopic surgery. Urology 42:2, 1993

6. Fishburne JI: Anesthesia for laparoscopy: considerations, complications and techniques. J Reprod Med 21:37, 1978

7. Keith L, Silver A, Becker M: Anesthesia for laparoscopy. J Reprod Med 12:227, 1974

8. Fitzgibbons R, Jr, Annibali R, Litke BS: Gallbladder and gallstone removal, open versus closed laparoscopy, and pneumoperitoneum. Am J Surg 165:497, 1993

9. Safran D, Sgambati S, Orlando R: Laparoscopy in high-risk cardiac patients. Surg Gynecol Obstet 176:548, 1993

10. Wahba RW, Mamazza J: Ventilatory requirements during laparoscopic cholecystectomy. Can J Anaesth 40:206, 1993

11. Ho HS, Saunders CJ, Corso FA et al: The effects of CO_2 pneumoperitoneum on hemodynamics in hemorrhaged animals. Surgery 114:381, 1993

12. Versichelen L, Serreyn R, Rolly G et al: Physiopathologic changes during anesthesia administration for gynecologic laparoscopy. J Reprod Med 29:697, 1984

13. Bardoczky GI, Engelman E, Levarlet M et al: Ventilatory effects of pneumoperitoneum monitored with continuous spirometry. Anaesthesia 48:309, 1993

14. Tolksdorf W, Strang CM, Schippers E et al: The effects of the carbon dioxide pneumoperitoneum in laparoscopic cholecystectomy on postoperative spontaneous respiration. Anaesthesist 41:199, 1992

15. Benhamou D, Simonneau G, Poynard T et al: Diaphragm function is not impaired by pneumoperitoneum after laparoscopy. Arch Surg 128:430, 1993

16. Crist DW, Gadacz TR: Complications of laparoscopic surgery. Surg Clin North Am 73:265, 1993

17. Whiston RJ, Eggers KA, Morris RW et al: Tension pneumothorax during laparoscopic cholecystectomy. Br J Surg 78:1325, 1991

18. Heddle RM, Platt AJ: Tension pneumothorax during laparoscopic cholecystectomy. Br J Surg 79:374, 1992

19. Moffa SM, Quinn JV, Slotman GJ: Hemodynamic effects of carbon dioxide pneumoperitoneum during mechanical ventilation and positive end-expiratory pressure. J Trauma 35:613, 1993

20. Motew M, Ivankovich AD, Bieniarz J et al: Cardiovascular effects and acid-base and blood gas changes during laparoscopy. Am J Obstet Gynecol 115:1002, 1973

21. Ishizaki Y, Bandai Y, Shimomura K et al: Changes in splanchnic blood flow and cardiovascular effects following peritoneal insufflation of carbon dioxide. Surg Endosc 7:420, 1993

22. Myles PS: Bradyarrhythmias and laparoscopy: a prospective study of heart rate changes with laparoscopy. Aust N Z J Obstet Gynaecol 31:171, 1991

23. Bard PA, Chen L: Subcutaneous emphysema associated with laparoscopy. Anesth Analg 71:101, 1990

24. Kalhan SB, Reaney JA, Collins RL: Pneumomediastinum and subcutaneous emphysema during laparoscopy. Cleve Clin J Med 57:639, 1990

25. Diakun TA: Carbon dioxide embolism: successful resuscitation with cardiopulmonary bypass. Anesthesiology 74:1151, 1991

26. Duncan C: Carbon dioxide embolism during laparoscopy: a case report. Aana J 60:139, 1992

27. Root B, Levy MN, Pollack S et al: Gas embolism death after laparoscopy delayed by "trapping" in portal circulation. Anesth Analg 57:232, 1978

28. Talamini MA, Gadacz TR: Laparoscopic equipment and instrumentation. p. 23. In Zucker K (ed): Surgical Laparoscopy. Quality Medical Publisher, St. Louis, 1991

29. Millard JA, Hill BB, Cook PS et al: Intermittent sequential pneumatic compression in prevention of venous stasis associated with pneumoperitoneum during laparoscopic cholecystectomy. Arch Surg 128:914, 1993

30. Mayol J, Vincent-Hamelin E, Sarmiento JM et al: Pulmonary embolism following laparoscopic cholecystectomy. Surg Endosc 8:214, 1994

31. Meltzer R, Chrostek C, Hoenig D et al: CO_2 vs N_2O insufflation for laparoscopic cholecystectomy. Surg Endosc 8:253, 1994

32. Leighton TA, Liu SY, Bongard FS: Comparative cardiopulmonary effects of carbon dioxide versus helium pneumoperitoneum. Surgery 113:527, 1993

33. Bailey RW: Complications of laparoscopic general surgery. p. 311. In Zucker K (ed): Surgical Laparoscopy. Quality Medical Publisher, St. Louis, 1991

34. Reich H: Laparoscopic treatment of extensive pelvic adhesions, including hydrosalpinx. J Reprod Med 32:736, 1987

35. Gagnon J, Poulin EC: Beware of the Trendelenburg position during prolonged laparoscopic procedures. Can J Surg 36:505, 1993

36. Romanowski L, Reich H, McGlynn F et al: Brachial plexus neuropathies after advanced laparoscopic surgery. Fertil Steril 60:729, 1993

37. al Hakim M, Katirji B: Femoral mononeuropathy induced by the lithotomy position: a report of 5 cases with a review of literature. Muscle Nerve 16:891, 1993

38. Kane MG, Krejs GJ: Complications of diagnostic laparoscopy in Dallas: a 7-year prospective study. Gastrointest Endosc 30:237, 1984

39. Lehmann-Willenbrock E, Riedel HH, Mecke H et al: Pelviscopy/laparoscopy and its complications in Germany, 1949-1988. J Reprod Med 37:671, 1992

40. Deziel DJ, Millikan KW, Economou SG et al: Complications of laparoscopic cholecystectomy: a national survey of 4,292 hospitals and an analysis of 77,604 cases. Am J Surg 165:9, 1993

41. Mintz M: Risks and prophylaxis in laparoscopy: a survey of 100,000 cases. J Reprod Med 18:269, 1977

42. Yuzpe AA: Pneumoperitoneum needle and trocar injuries in laparoscopy. A survey on possible contributing factors and prevention. J Reprod Med 35:485, 1990

43. Baadsgaard SE, Bille S, Egeblad K: Major vascular injury during gynecologic laparoscopy. Report of a case and review of published cases. Acta Obstet Gynecol Scand 68:283, 1989

44. Colver RM: Laparoscopy: basic technique, instrumentation, and complications. Surg Laparosc Endosc 2:35, 1992

45. Sia-Kho E, Kelly RE: Urinary drainage bag distention: an indication of bladder injury during laparoscopy. J Clin Anesth 4:346, 1992

46. Kurtz BR, Daniell JF, Spaw AT: Incarcerated incisional hernia after laparoscopy. A case report. J Reprod Med 38:643, 1993

47. Baird DR, Wilson JP, Mason EM et al: An early review of 800 laparoscopic cholecystectomies at a university-affiliated community teaching hospital. Am Surg 58:206, 1992

48. Kleppinger RK: Laparoscopy at a community hospital: an analysis of 4,300 cases. J Reprod Med 19:353, 1977

49. Peters, Gibbons GD, Innes JT et al: Complications of laparoscopic cholecystectomy. Surgery 110:769, 1991

50. Hass BE, Schrager RE: Small bowel obstruction due to Richter's hernia after laparoscopic procedures. J Laparoendosc Surg 3:421, 1993

51. Moossa AR, Easter DW, Van Sonnenberg E et al: Laparoscopic injuries to the bile duct. A cause for concern. Ann Surg 215:203, 1992

52. Peterson HB, Ory HW, Greenspan JR et al: Deaths associated with laparoscopic sterilization by unipolar electrocoagulating devices, 1978 and 1979. Am J Obstet Gynecol 139:141, 1981

53. Genyk YS, Keller FS, Halpern NB: Hepatic artery pseudoaneurysm and hemobilia following laser laparoscopic cholecystectomy. Surg Endosc 8:201, 1994

54. Berry SM, Ose KJ, Bell RH et al: Thermal injury of the posterior duodenum during laparoscopic cholecystectomy. Surg Endosc 8:197, 1994

55. Voyles CR, Tucker RD: Unrecognized hazards of surgical electrodes passed through metal suction-irrigation devices. Surg Endosc 8:185, 1993

56. Hunter JG: Laser or electrocautery for laparoscopic cholecystectomy? Am J Surg 161:345, 1991

57. Voyles CR, Petro AB, Meena AL et al: A practical approach to laparoscopic cholecystectomy. Am J Surg 161:365, 1991

58. Miner DW, Levine RL: Microbiologic effects of atmospheric conditions used in operative laparoscopy. J Reprod Med 38:531, 1993

59. Sotrel G, Hirsch E, Edelin KC: Necrotizing fasciitis following diagnostic laparoscopy. Obstet Gynecol 62:67s, 1983

60. Nelson MT, Nakashima M, Mulvihill SJ: How secure are laparoscopically placed clips? An in vitro and in vivo study. Arch Surg 127:718, 1992

61. Stewart L, Hunter J, Oddsdottir M et al: Prevention of bile duct injuries during laparoscopic cholecystectomy. Ann Surg, 1995, In press

62. Wolfe BM, Gardiner BN, Leary BF et al: Endoscopic cholecystectomy. An analysis of complications. Arch Surg 126:1192, 1991

63. Ferguson CM, Rattner DW, Warshaw AL: Bile duct injury in laparoscopic cholecystectomy. Surg Laparosc Endosc 2:1, 1992

64. Woods MS, Traverso LW, Kozarek RA et al: Characteristics of biliary tract complications during laparoscopic cholecystectomy: a multi-institutional study. Am J Surg 167:27, 1994

65. Rossi RL, Schirmer WJ, Braasch JW et al: Laparoscopic bile duct injuries. Risk factors, recognition, and repair. Arch Surg 127:596, 1992

66. Hunter JG: Avoidance of bile duct injury during laparoscopic cholecystectomy. Am J Surg 162:71, 1991

67. Sackier JM, Berci G, Phillips E et al: The role of cholangiography in laparoscopic cholecystectomy. Arch Surg 126:1021, 1991

68. Flowers JL, Zucker KA, Graham SM et al: Laparoscopic cholangiography. Results and indications. Ann Surg 215:209, 1992

69. Soper NJ: Laparoscopic cholecystectomy. Curr Probl Surg 28:581, 1991

70. MacFadyen B, Jr, Arregui ME, Corbitt J, Jr et al: Complications of laparoscopic herniorrhaphy. Surg Endosc 7:155, 1993

71. Fitzgibbons R, Annibali R, Litke B et al: A multicentered clinical trial on laparoscopic inguinal hernia repair: preliminary results. Surg Endosc 7:115, 1993

72. Wheeler KH: Laparoscopic inguinal herniorrhaphy with mesh: an 18-month experience. J Laparoendosc Surg 3:345, 1993

73. Woods S, Polglase A: Ilioinguinal nerve entrapment from laparoscopic hernia repair. Aust N Z J Surg 63:823, 1993

74. Kraus MA: Nerve injury during laparoscopic inguinal hernia repair. Surg Laparosc Endosc 3:342, 1993

75. Arregui ME, Navarrete J, Davis CJ et al: Laparoscopic inguinal herniorrhaphy. Surg Clin North Am 73:513, 1993

76. Attwood SE, Hill AD, Murphy PG et al: A prospective randomized trial of laparoscopic versus open appendectomy. Surgery 112:497, 1992

77. Cox MR, McCall JL, Wilson TG et al: Laparoscopic appendicectomy: a prospective analysis. Aust N Z J Surg 63:840, 1993

78. Schroder DM, Lathrop JC, Lloyd LR et al: Laparoscopic appendectomy for acute appendicitis: is there really any benefit? Am Surg 59:541, 1993

79. Vallina VL, Velasco JM, McCulloch CS: Laparoscopic versus conventional appendectomy. Ann Surg 218:685, 1993

80. Tate JJ, Chung SC, Dawson J et al: Conventional versus laparoscopic surgery for acute appendicitis. Br J Surg 80:761, 1993

81. Lewis FR, Holcroft JW, Boey J et al: Appendicitis: a critical review of diagnosis and treatment in 1,000 cases. Arch Surg 110:677, 1975

82. Pier A, Gotz F, Bacher C: Laparoscopic appendectomy in 625 cases: from innovation to routine. Surg Laparosc Endosc 1:8, 1991

83. Falk PM, Beart R, Jr, Wexner SD et al: Laparoscopic colectomy: a critical appraisal. Dis Colon Rectum 36:28, 1993

84. Monson JR, Darzi A, Carey PD et al: Prospective evaluation of laparoscopic-assisted colectomy in an unselected group of patients [see comments]. Lancet 340:831, 1992

85. Schlinkert RT: Laparoscopic-assisted right hemicolectomy. Dis Colon Rectum 34:1030, 1991

86. Wexner SD, Johansen OB, Nogueras JJ et al: Laparoscopic total abdominal colectomy. A prospective trial. Dis Colon Rectum 35:651, 1992

87. Wexner SD, Johansen OB: Laparoscopic bowel resection: advantages and limitations. Ann Med 24:105, 1992

88. Phillips EH, Franklin M, Carroll BJ et al: Laparoscopic colectomy. Ann Surg 216:703, 1992

89. Alexander RJ, Jaques BC, Mitchell KG: Laparoscopically assisted colectomy and wound recurrence. Lancet 341:249, 1993

90. Walsh DC, Wattchow DA, Wilson TG: Subcutaneous metastases after laparoscopic resection of malignancy. Aust N Z J Surg 63:563, 1993

9

▸ Learning Laparoscopic Surgery

L. W. Way

S. Bhoyrul

T. Mori

VIDEO ENDOSCOPIC SURGERY IS A NEW WAY OF OPERATING THAT specific problems that must be identified and overcome. Many of the required skills are not used in open surgery. The early recognition that the rate of complications correlates with the number of procedures done by the surgeon[1] has highlighted the need for formal training in laparoscopic surgery. No consensus has been reached, however, on what constitutes adequate training. This chapter discusses training methods and goals based on reports of others and our experience at the Advanced Videoscopic Training Center, University of California, San Francisco, Medical Center.

Training in laparoscopic surgery includes didactic instruction, in vitro training in simulators, and operating on animals and patients. Each kind of training has its merits and limitations, which must be considered when embarking on a training program. Also, in some centers, the approach to training for surgical residents who need an overview of laparoscopic procedures and techniques differs slightly from training for experienced surgeons wishing to develop a specific laparoscopic practice. Some evidence indicates that it may not be necessary for specialized surgeons to learn how to perform basic procedures (e.g., the laparoscopic cholecystectomy) before learning how to perform a more advanced procedure. It has been shown that the ability to perform a laparoscopic cholecystectomy does not confer the level of skill for more advanced procedures, such as the colon resection,[2] and also that colon resection can be taught without prior experience of laparoscopic cholecystectomy.[3] Although specialized surgeons can be taught to perform advanced procedures without experience of the more basic ones, we are concerned that the complication rates (shown to be related to the total number of procedures done[1]) will be higher for these surgeons when compared with surgeons with a greater experience of laparoscopic surgery. We therefore recommend that all surgeons be trained in simpler laparoscopic procedures before performing more difficult ones.

Didactic Instruction

Didactic instruction occurs in various settings: during training courses, postgraduate courses, and meetings of surgical societies. The two components are general instruction and specific procedural training.

The general component should cover familiarization with the instruments, especially the principles of using and troubleshooting the imaging system; principles of operative techniques, especially trocar placement; exposure of the operating field; and principles of intracorporeal suturing. This instruction is necessary before specific procedures are attempted, especially procedures requiring the use of two hands (see Ch. 3) and intracorporeal suturing.

Training surgeons to perform specific procedures should include a brief explanation of the key steps of the procedure and showing videotapes. The material that should be presented on these tapes and suggestions for the surgeon producing these tapes are summarized below. The key steps in the procedure should be pointed out while the proper instruments are discussed (e.g., electrosurgery, dissectors, and graspers). Videotapes should be available for students to review at their convenience. The major complications and their avoidance should be covered. Videotapes of complications or "near complications" have a great impact.

Steps in Producing an Educational Video

1. Plan the video and script beforehand. Know your audience.
2. Aim for a final edited version of 5 to 10 minutes per operative procedure.
3. Use either super VHS, high 8, or Betamax tapes to shoot the original video.
4. Introduce the goals of the tape with a narration or graphics.
5. When recording the tape, the camera operator should deliberately record footage that would help reorient the viewer (e.g., it is useful to have a broad perspective before the details of an anastomosis are shown).
6. If sound is involved, it is preferable to have the tape narrated by the surgeon rather than a professional narrator. Music is difficult to use and may be counterproductive. If in doubt don't use it.
7. Professional involvement or broadcast quality equipment is useful, especially for production and editing.

In Vitro Training

The first step is practice in a trainer, an inexpensive box with ports for instruments and the scope. Many trainers are commercially available, ranging in design from plastic boxes with holes for trocar placement to those with a small video camera built in (Fig. 9-1), so that they may be connected directly to a TV monitor without having to borrow a camera and light source from the operating room. The latter design is more convenient for the surgeon wishing to practice in his or her office.

In vitro training can be a valuable supplement to experience in live animals and humans in several areas. First, it is useful for establishing the team interaction between surgeon, camera operator, and assistant.[4] It is the best time to learn how to use the camera. We use in vitro trainers mainly to teach intra-

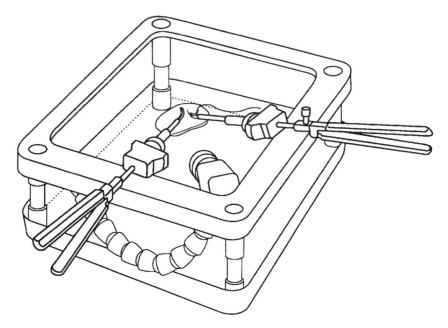

Fig. 9-1. An inexpensive laparoscopic trainer device that allows the surgeon to practice skills (e.g., suturing) in his or her office. The camera may be connected directly to a TV monitor. Note the absence of a light source or laparoscope.

corporeal suturing skills and live animals to teach operative surgery. Most of the students can acquire the basic skills (i.e., placing and tying a suture) in about 2 hours. Progress beyond that varies between surgeons and is influenced by the frequency of practice. An experienced instructor should do the teaching because many steps (e.g., mounting the needle in the needle holder, laying out the suture, and best use of the camera) are not intuitive and differ from those in open surgery. Goals during the suturing should be to complete the prescribed knots within the standard times, as seen in Chapter 4. In countries where live animals are less easily available for training, some centers practice dissecting technique and simulated operations on fresh slaughterhouse organs in an in vitro trainer.[5]

Use of Animals for Training

Operating on live pigs (we use female Hampshire pigs; average weight 60 lbs) is extremely useful for developing skills, trying out new procedures, and gaining experience with new and unfamiliar instruments. Approval must be obtained from the institution's animal use committee. The cost of running and supporting an animal care facility usually limits this activity to academic centers. The cost of operating on a pig, which includes the cost of the animal, anesthesia, and veterinary support, is approximately $500. This excludes the cost of the laparoscopic instruments, which can usually be salvaged from the hospital operating room or obtained as a donation from manufacturers.

In general, the pig is a good model for acquiring skills such as trocar placement, exposure, and the appropriate use of gravity, traction, and countertraction. Other important skills, such as two-handed dissection, intracorporeal suturing, use of mechanical stapling and anastomosis devices, and dealing with complications such as bleeding and bowel perforation can also be learned during operations on pigs.

Training for Specific Procedures in the Pig

The pig is a good model for the surgeon to practice dissecting the gallbladder from the liver bed during cholecystectomy, but no animal really mimics the anatomy of Calot's triangle enough to be a good model for the human operation. This limitation has to be borne in mind when transferring experience gained in pigs to humans, because the most serious technical complications of cholecystectomy occur from mistakes during the dissection of Calot's triangle (see Ch. 8). Furthermore, the cystic duct of the pig is too small for transcystic common bile duct exploration. Anatomic differences also make the pig a poor model for appendectomy, right hemicolectomy, and hysterectomy.

The pig is an excellent model for operations on the upper gastrointestinal tract. We use it for antireflux procedures, vagotomy, Heller cardiomyotomy, pyloroplasty, gastrectomy, gastrostomy, jejunostomy, cholecystojejunostomy, and gastrojejunostomy. Experience in these operations in pigs is relevant to the same operations in humans. The pig is also a good model for laparoscopic-assisted anterior resection of the colon, although the absence of fat in the mesentery makes the mesenteric dissection easier in pigs than in humans. The pig is also a reasonable model for laparoscopic transperitoneal hernia repair. The anatomy is not too dissimilar; the main difference is that the pig has two inferior epigastric arteries. The procedure itself can be easily performed in pigs. Preperitoneal hernia repairs and other preperitoneal procedures are more difficult to simulate in pigs because their peritoneum is thinner than in humans. Therefore, it has a tendency to tear, which leads to loss of the pneumopreperitoneum. Splenectomy may be performed in pigs, but the pig spleen has a different shape and is more mobile than the human spleen.

Method and Limitations of Training in the Animal Laboratory

Animal training most often takes place during formal courses, usually organized by academic institutions or instrument companies. Three students per pig, with students rotating as surgeon, camera operator, and assistant, is a good arrangement at the start. It is ideal if the three students come from the same institution and plan to operate as a team after completing the course. One instructor is assigned to each group of three students. The instructors must have first-hand experience that makes them experts. Over the period of the course, the students should be exposed to different instructors and thus to different operating styles and techniques. Whether this method of training translates to improved performance in the human operating room is yet to be shown. Feedback from course participants has been positive.

The major limitation of animal training courses is that students cannot really gain enough experience to perform the more difficult operations, such as fundoplication, on humans. Even after a three-day course on one procedure (laparoscopic cholecystectomy), some students remain unable to complete the procedure satisfactorily as judged by supervisors.[6] No data are available to indicate how much experience is truly required to bring performance to an acceptable threshold. In an experimental model, we have found considerable variation in the surgical skills of individual laparoscopic surgeons.[7] One or two courses may be insufficient for many surgeons. There is a growing belief that permanent training facilities are needed where surgeons can train regularly until they reach a point where they are fully prepared to perform technically difficult procedures in humans. A better understanding of the nature of surgical skills and how to measure them is also needed.

The Role of Technology in Training

New technology promises to improve the effectiveness of training programs and the capabilities of surgeons in the operating room. For example, virtual reality trainers (Ch. 10) may facilitate the objective assessment and training of laparoscopic surgeons and decrease dependence on animal models.

Furthermore, manufacturers are attempting to produce devices (most of which are still experimental) that simplify more difficult tasks, such as suturing. If successful, this should allow more surgeons to perform advanced laparoscopic procedures.

Training in Humans

Several studies have shown that the rate of complications is greater during the early part of a surgeon's experience (see Ch. 8), which raises serious questions about the ethics of exposing patients to these increased risks. Essentially, in present practice, the surgeon's first 10 patients become part of his training program. The most obvious ways to deal with this issue are to increase the amount of practice in laboratory exercises and to provide greater supervision during the transition to human surgery. The practical obstacles to such an expanded training program are substantial, however.

The surgeon should be phased into performing human cases by assisting experienced colleagues and then being proctored by these colleagues. Eventually, training during residency programs must reach a point where the graduates are proficient.[8,9] The situation at present consists of a faculty who are still learning and a volume of experience that leaves the graduate on the steepest part of the learning curve. Furthermore, it is still only vaguely perceived just how much training and supervised experience is adequate. This is currently the focus of research.[7] We believe that it is possible to make objective analyses of technical performance during laparoscopic surgery. If so, the data could be used to gauge progress during training and to establish an index of competency to operate on humans.

The issue of privileging criteria for laparoscopic surgery has been addressed by various interested parties. The Society of American Gastrointestinal Endoscopic Surgeons (SAGES) and the Society for Surgeons of the Alimentary Tract (SSAT) made similar recommendations:

1. Laparoscopic surgeons should be trained general surgeons who have privileges to perform the open procedure.
2. They should be credentialed in diagnostic laparoscopy.
3. They should first receive formal training in laparoscopic surgery in a course with didactic and practical instruction.
4. They must be assisted in their initial clinical experience by an experienced surgeon.

In the United States, the responsibility for setting privileging criteria rests with the surgical staff of individual hospitals. The extent to which hospitals have really come to grips with this subject has not been systematically studied, but anecdotal information suggests that the SAGES and SSAT recommendations have not been fully implemented in many hospitals. Furthermore, the most critical and difficult step—effective proctoring—seems to be especially prone to compromise.

Finally, some important conclusions were reached in a study of predictors of laparoscopic complications *after* the surgeons attended a training course.[10] First, the risk of complications after a course was more than three times higher in surgeons who did not seek additional training. Second, the likelihood of complications could be decreased by attending the course with a partner from the same practice and undertaking the new laparoscopic procedures as a group rather than as an individual. Third, performing the operations with the same assistant (the buddy system) also reduced the likelihood of complications. These findings highlight the need for continuing education after a course and also point to practical ways in which the incidence of laparoscopic complications may be reduced.

Conclusion

Laparoscopic surgery demands a higher level of skill than open surgery. Learning these new techniques should begin during residency and should progress through in vitro training, didactic instruction, experience in animal models, and assisting and proctoring in human cases. Technologic advances will undoubtedly have an influence on training and may lessen the skill required for acceptable performance. Objective assessment of surgical skills as an aid to training is needed.

References

1. The Southern Surgeons Club: A prospective analysis of 1518 laparoscopic cholecystectomies. N Engl J Med 324:1073, 1991
2. Grundfest WS: Credentialing in an era of change. JAMA 270:2725, 1993
3. Milsom JW, Lavery IC, Church JM et al: Use of laparoscopic techniques in colorectal surgery. Preliminary study. Dis Colon Rectum 37:215, 1994

4. Sackier JM, Berci G, Paz-Partlow M: A new training device for laparoscopic cholecystectomy. Surg Endosc 5:158, 1991

5. Watson DI, Majeed AW, Johnson AG: Simulated laparoscopic Nissen fundoplication. Minimally Invasive Therapy 3:147, 1994

6. Hunter JG, Sackier JM, Berci G: Training in laparoscopic cholecystectomy. Quantifying the learning curve. Surg Endosc 8(1):28, 1994

7. Bhoyrul S, Tendick F, Mori T, Way LW: An analysis of perceptual motor skills of laparoscopic surgeons. Surg Endosc 8:534, 1994

8. Bailey RW, Imbembo AL, Zucker KA: Establishment of a laparoscopic cholecystectomy training program. Am Surg 57:231, 1991.

9. Schrimer BD, Edge SB, Dix J, Miller AD: Incorporation of laparoscopy into a surgical endoscopy training program. Am J Surg 163:46, 1992

10. See WA, Cooper CS, Fisher RJ: Predictors of laparoscopic complications after formal training in laparoscopic surgery. JAMA 270:2689, 1993

10

▶ Future of Laparoscopic Surgery

F. Tendick
T. Mori
L. W. Way

ADVANCES IN LAPAROSCOPIC SURGERY TOOK PLACE WHEN IMPROVEMENTS in surgical skill and technology increased the scope of beneficial procedures. About 80 percent of abdominal operations theoretically could be performed laparoscopically. Feasibility, however, does not ensure benefit to the patient. In particular, laparoscopic surgery may not be a good choice when there are better alternatives or when the procedure is too technically demanding. This highlights the need in many situations for controlled clinical trials to evaluate the benefits and drawbacks of a particular procedure. In a specialty that has been patient driven and industry sponsored, this has not always been the case. Improved medical management may make some laparoscopic procedures obsolete. For example, laparoscopic vagotomy was initially an excellent alternative to long-term drug therapy for chronic duodenal ulcer, because it compared well in overall cost and results.[1,2] However, vagotomy is virtually obsolete now as a treatment for peptic ulcer, because it is known that the disease can usually be cured by eradicating *Helicobacter pylori* infection.[3,4]

Several prospective randomized trials have compared laparoscopic with conventional operations for appendectomy and inguinal hernia repair. The results show that the laparoscopic approach provides additional diagnostic information, shortens hospital stay, and decreases postoperative discomfort. The disadvantages are the need for general anesthesia, a longer operating time, and higher costs. Whether to do the operation laparoscopically should be decided by balancing these benefits and risks. Although laparoscopic (assisted) colectomy is technically feasible, its efficacy and safety as a curative cancer operation remain unproved.

Some procedures cannot be performed laparoscopically, because access to the surgical site (exposure) is inadequate or because the procedure is so technically difficult that the operating time is too long and the risk of complications too high. Technical advances could theoretically overcome these problems.

Exposure

The three major areas where technical advances may be expected to widen the scope of laparoscopic procedures are improvements in exposure (e.g., gasless laparoscopy), retroperitoneal and mediastinal access, and laparoscopic access to the lumen of hollow organs.

Gasless Laparoscopy

Creation of a space in which to operate (i.e., exposure) plays a vital role in minimally invasive surgery. Several methods of mechanically lifting the abdominal wall eliminate the need for a pneumoperitoneum.[5,6] They all depend on devices that can be anchored to the abdominal wall and lifted upward, including an L-shaped hook, a helical device, and a subcutaneous wire. The upward traction allows air to enter the abdomen through the port sites.

With these point sources of lift, however, the resulting abdominal space resembles a tent raised by a center pole instead of one with a dome (as with a pneumoperitoneum.) The viscera remain crowded, so exposure is compromised and even simple operations such as cholecystectomy can be more difficult than usual. If the area of retraction can be expanded, however, the force of the retraction would be more diffuse and less traumatic, and the space created would have a broad ceiling. Because of their drawbacks, current systems are largely limited to procedures on the lower abdomen.

Gasless exposure, however, has many potential benefits. The complications of pneumoperitoneum would be avoided. Airtight valves would be unnecessary in the cannulas, so conventional surgical instruments could be used. And more than one instrument could be inserted through a single site, avoiding the need for multiple trocar incisions.

One solution might be a cage or skeleton that stretches the abdominal wall from the inside, or a balloon that displaces the organs and abdominal wall but still allows surgical maneuvers. New ways of exposure could drastically change the instrumentation and techniques in minimally invasive surgery.

Retroperitoneal and Mediastinal Access

Improved methods of exposure allow new procedures to be performed. For example, laparoscopic antireflux procedures were facilitated by instruments (e.g., the liver retractor) that simplified exposure of the gastroesophageal junction.[9] Similarly, advances in instrumentation and techniques that expose the retroperitoneal space or mediastinum should further widen the range of minimally invasive procedures.

Laparoscopic surgery of the kidney and the adrenal gland is currently performed by a transperitoneal approach.[10–12] A hydraulic balloon for dissecting the retroperitoneal space has been developed, making it possible to work in the retroperitoneum without entering the abdominal cavity.[13,14] Using low-pressure insufflation of the retroperitoneal space, intra-abdominal organs are pushed aside, so the retroperitoneal organs can be seen. The risk of injuring the intra-abdominal viscera with the trocars is low.

Refinements have also made it feasible to expose the abdominal aorta and iliac vessels.[15] Para-aortic lymph node dissection for gynecologic and urologic malignancies is possible, but the role of laparoscopic operations in the management of these diseases is yet to be fully evaluated.[16] Aortobifemoral bypass has also been successfully performed through a retroperitoneal minimally invasive approach.[17] The aortic anastomosis was performed through a small abdominal incision (i.e., it was a laparoscopic-assisted operation). Patients with aortoiliac vascular disease presumably would benefit from laparoscopic solutions to their problems, because they so often have concomitant cardiopulmonary disorders. Laser tissue welding[18] might also make laparoscopic vascular surgery easier and safer.

Mediastinal procedures have been performed by minimally invasive techniques, including procedures for esophageal motor disorders,[19,20] esophagectomy for benign and malignant disease,[21,22] mediastinal lymph node sampling and dissection,[23] biopsy and resection of mediastinal tumors,[24–26] and vascular procedures.[27,28] Thoracoscopic approaches to the mediastinum have been facilitated by anesthetic techniques (e.g., differential lung ventilation) and improved surgical instruments (e.g., lung retractor). The longer operating times and inability to inflate the lung periodically, however, sometimes results in prolonged lung collapse and postoperative pulmonary complications. This served as an impetus to develop a mediastinoscope with dissecting capabilities.[29] To date, mediastinoscopy has proved to be much less versatile than thoracoscopy for diagnostic and therapeutic procedures.[23] Still, mediastinoscopy has much promise.

Thoracoscopic vascular procedures by minimally invasive surgery, such as interruption of patent ductus arteriosus, have been performed mainly in children. Although these have been successful, the instruments could be improved substantially (e.g., clip applier for specific use and shorter instruments).[30,31] Many surgeons anticipate that advances in devices would make minimally invasive surgery feasible even on the heart and major vessels.

Intraluminal Access

The lumen of a hollow organ is a potential area for minimally invasive surgery. In fact, laparoscopic access to the lumen is now possible for organs previously accessible only by endoscopy or a large enterotomy.

Surgery within the lumen of an organ (intraluminal surgery) has been facilitated greatly by the advent of specially designed cannulas that puncture the organ with a needle and then expand radially to the functional size. When the cannula is removed, only a small defect in the wall of the viscus remains, which can be closed with one or two sutures,[32] obviating the need for an enterotomy for exposure. The wide range of instruments available to the laparoscopic surgeon allows various procedures to be performed (including suturing) within the lumen — much more than is possible through fiber-optic endoscopes.

The first useful example of intraluminal laparoscopic surgery was in the treatment of pancreatic pseudocysts. Cannulas are introduced into the lumen of the stomach under laparoscopic control as the gastric lumen is inflated with carbon dioxide (instilled through a nasogastric tube). Surgery can then be performed by instruments introduced into the lumen through the cannulas under the view of a 5-mm laparoscope introduced through one of the cannulas. Another imaging approach is to use a flexible gastroscope passed perorally, but it is very difficult to orient the view properly, so this approach is unsatisfactory except for the simplest procedures.

To drain a pancreatic pseudocyst, an incision is made through the back wall of the stomach into the cyst. The incision can be made the same size as in open surgery, hemostasis with cautery is excellent, and the cyst contents can be debrided thoroughly under direct vision. Partial excision of the gastric wall for benign and malignant lesions,[33] excision of broad-based cecal polyps, and a transduodenal or transgastric approach to a sphincterotomy of the papilla of Vater have been performed laparoscopically.[34] Upper gastrointestinal bleeding may also be treated this way when endoscopic intervention has failed. Gastric varices, which are difficult to manage endoscopically, might be treated by this method, although no experience has yet been reported. Many other procedures are conceivable.

Intraluminal surgery may also be of use in organs inaccessible to conventional endoscopy. For example, small bowel enteroscopy is possible using these methods.

Similar techniques have been used for in utero fetal surgery (i.e., fetoscopic surgery). Open fetal surgery has been successfully performed for serious malformations, such as congenital diaphragmatic hernia, cystic adenomatoid malformation, obstructive uropathy, and massive sacrococcygeal teratoma.[35,36] Prenatal repair of these lesions presently requires open hysterotomy, which may result in preterm labor.[37] The only clinical application of fetoscopic surgery to date has been cord ligation for twin-to-twin transfusion.[38,39] If techniques can be refined, however, fetoscopic surgery may be used for these other malformations, such as cleft lip and palate and neural tube defects.[40]

Perception and Dexterity Enhancement

The set-up for laparoscopic surgery presents a challenge to the surgeon's perceptual motor skills. One must rely on an image of the surgical space that is degraded by the optics, camera, and display processing through which it passes. Tactile sensation is lost. Kinesthetic feedback of the forces exerted on tissue is reduced by friction of instruments in the cannula. Dexterity is diminished by the fulcrum effect of the instruments at the point where the cannula passes through the abdominal wall.

There are two ways to overcome these obstacles. Training (see Ch. 9) can teach the skills necessary to work as effectively as possible. Better instruments can restore some of the image quality, sensation, and dexterity that are missing in current instruments.

Enhanced Vision

One of the most significant limitations in laparoscopic surgery results from the compromise in viewing conditions with conventional video endoscopes.[41] This is primarily due to the lack of stereopsis with a single endoscope image. Stereopsis is the visual depth acuity that the brain interprets from the disparity between the images received by the two eyes (binocular disparity). Useful monoscopic depth cues are present, however, even when only a single image is available. For example, the experienced surgeon can learn to gauge distances roughly by using perspective cues (e.g., the change of apparent object size with distance), variations in reflected light with the distance of surfaces from the light source, and parallax (i.e., the apparent side-to-side motion of objects) from endoscope motion. Positions can be confirmed by instrument contact. Nevertheless, in tasks requiring the most accurate depth perception, stereopsis is the most robust depth cue.[42]

To restore stereoscopic vision in laparoscopic surgery, several manufacturers have developed stereoscopic (three-dimensional) laparoscopes. The common way to create a stereo image is to use two optical paths within the laparoscope tube.[43] The paired images project onto two charge-coupled device (CCD) cameras and are displayed alternately on a stereo display monitor. The images are separated for viewing by circularly polarizing filters used on the display and on glasses worn by the viewer. As the left and right images alternate on the display at a rate of 60 or 120 times a second, the active filter on the display switches polarization in synchrony. Each of the viewer's eyes sees only the image intended for it when the active filter polarization matches the polarization of that eye's lens in the viewing glasses. Another kind of display uses active shutters on the glasses, switched in synchrony with the monitor.

It is important to understand that a stereo laparoscope must create binocular disparity with optics that image two laterally offset views. Stereo optics and display methods have been developed, in addition to those described above, that create true binocular disparity. However, one should be wary of systems that claim to be stereo or three dimensional but use depth cues other than stereopsis, or create false disparity by taking a single image and shifting it laterally for each eye. These systems may not provide the accurate perception of depth afforded by stereopsis.

Many difficulties are associated with the design of a stereo viewing system. For example, the disparity between the stereo pair views, which produces the stereoscopic effect, is limited because the separation of the two optical paths cannot exceed the diameter of the endoscope. This separation is about one tenth of the average human interocular distance of 65 mm. Human stereopsis is good within a 1-meter viewing distance, so it might be expected from geometry that stereo endoscopic viewing would be effective at one tenth of this distance, or 10 cm. Several other factors influence stereo disparity, however. Because the resolution of video monitors is much lower than that of the eye, disparity is limited. Endoscope field of view, video monitor size, and viewer distance from the monitor affect the display magnification, which can increase effective disparity. No published data show the effects of these parameters in typical laparoscopic tasks.

The two optical paths must be precisely aligned and oriented to allow maximum disparity and reduce viewer fatigue.[44] This is difficult to achieve, because even thermal expansion of the endoscope can alter alignment enough to create a noticeable effect.[43]

The display of stereoscopic images is also a challenge. Accommodation (i.e., focusing of the eye) and convergence (i.e., inward rotation of the eyes to view near objects) cues, important aspects of normal viewing, cannot be duplicated in present display systems.[44] Polarized filtering reduces image brightness by more than 50 percent. Neither the filters nor the phosphors in the cathode ray tube (CRT) display can switch instantaneously, so it is possible to get "crosstalk," where the right eye image is partly seen by the left eye and vice versa. These problems can cause viewer fatigue.

Early evaluations of stereo endoscopes have demonstrated benefits, particularly in tasks, such as grasping a loose end of a suture, that demand good depth perception (F. Tendick, unpublished results 1993). Nevertheless, performance of ordinary tasks with stereo endoscopes is still not as good as with normal vision (i.e., as in open surgery).[45] It will be important to study stereo systems to determine whether and in what respects they confer advantages over the best monoscopic systems.

Other visual enhancements could also help. Currently, the laparoscope acts as the only light source, and areas far from the laparoscope tip may not receive enough illumination to produce a good image. A second light source (e.g., attached to a cannula) could provide additional light.

The human eye is better at perceiving contrast than gradual changes in brightness. Digital contrast enhancement of the video image may help the display of important features in a cluttered environment, such as a suture against a background of tissue mottled with blood.

Enhanced Dexterity

To understand how improved instrumentation could enhance surgical dexterity, one must first understand the mechanics governing dexterity.

To describe the position and orientation of an object in space, six coordinates are necessary. Three specify position—the location of an airplane in flight, for example. Three more are needed to specify orientation, typically, coordinates of rotation about orthogonal axes—for example, the roll, pitch, and yaw of an airplane.

The smallest number of coordinates that can describe the motion of a mechanical system is specified as its *degrees of freedom*. When the motion of an object is constrained, it may have fewer than 6 degrees of freedom. For example, a hinged door has only 1 degree of freedom: rotation about the hinge axis. Complex systems may have more than 6 degrees of freedom. The human arm has seven: three rotations (flexion-extension, abduction-adduction, and medial-lateral rotation) about the shoulder, one (flexion-extension) at the elbow, and three (flexion-extension, abduction-adduction, and pronation-supination) in the wrist and forearm. The human hand has over 20 degrees of freedom.

When a system such as the arm and hand has more than 6 degrees of freedom, many ways to produce the same action may be possible. For example, one can rest the forearm on a stable surface to reduce tremor while making a precise movement with finger control of an instrument. This is possible because the many degrees of freedom in the hand and wrist allow a range of forearm posture independent of the instrument motion controlled by the fingers.

When a system has fewer than 6 degrees of freedom, some motions are impossible. The major source of difficulty in the use of laparoscopic instruments is reduction in the degrees of freedom caused by the fixed fulcrum at the abdominal wall. The surgeon can move the instrument handle up and down, left and right, and in and out, and can rotate it about its long axis. This constitutes only 4 degrees of freedom. The resulting motion of the instrument tip inside the abdomen allows positioning of the tip anywhere within the limit of the instrument length. What is lost is the ability to orient the instrument tip. A given position inside the abdomen may be approached only from the direction defined by the axis between that position and the point of entry through the abdominal wall (Fig. 10-1). No other orientations except rotation about that axis are possible.

Consequently, maneuvers that require reorientation of instruments are most affected by the reduced degrees of freedom. Some tasks, such as stapling, may be improved with instruments capable of flexing at the tip. For techniques requiring complex movements with two instruments, particularly knot tying, instruments with more complex designs may well be beneficial.[41]

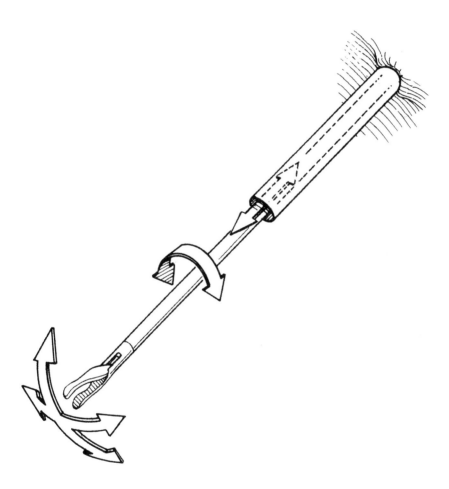

Fig. 10-1. Because of the fixed fulcrum at the abdominal wall, laparoscopic instruments are limited to 4 degrees of freedom.

Such instruments should permit at least two additional rotational degrees of freedom of the instrument tip. The major difficulty will be to design the instrument so there is simple and intuitive control of the additional motions.

Laparoscopic instruments have other shortcomings. Tactile sensation is lost because the surgeon's hand cannot palpate tissues. Friction in the cannulae reduces the kinesthetic sense of the resistance of tissues to forces exerted by instruments. The surgeon has no place to rest the wrist or arm to reduce tremor when holding laparoscopic instruments.

A possible technical solution is teleoperation (or telemanipulation), "the extension of a person's sensing and manipulation capability to a remote location."[46] In teleoperative laparoscopic surgery, the "remote" site is inside the patient's body. The surgeon could be in the operating room or far away (i.e., in a different city). The surgeon holds a master controller that transmits hand motions to the instrument and receives force and tactile information in return (Fig. 10-2). The slave manipulator inside the patient mimics the surgeon's motions and senses the forces that result from contact with tissue. A computer handles the flow of data between master and slave. If the surgeon is far from the patient, a high-speed communication link (e.g., via satellite) is necessary.

Teleoperation technology has existed for decades for nuclear material processing, undersea work, and space exploration. Some of the problems faced in laparoscopic surgery have been solved by researchers in these areas; others must be solved specifically for surgical applications. In particular, teleoperative surgery requires dexterity on a smaller scale than in past applications.

Because the fulcrum at the cannula allows only 4 degrees of freedom, a slave manipulator should have at least an additional 2 degrees of freedom inside the abdomen. A robotic manipulator can control the motions outside the patient's body.[47] A multijointed finger or a flexible snake-like manipulator can then extend motion inside the body.[48] A major engineering problem in creating a laparoscopic slave is activation of the degrees of freedom inside the abdomen. This requires either tiny actuators that fit through the cannula or a means to transmit forces from larger actuators into the body by cable, pneumatic, or hydraulic transmission. Innovative actuator technologies, including shape memory alloys (memory metals) and contractile polymers, may make centimeter-scale actuators feasible.[49] Safety will be an essential issue in the design of slave manipulators. Both hardware and software mechanisms will be necessary to prevent dangerous motions.[50]

Forces (and torques) of contact with tissue must be measured in all six coordinate directions in the slave manipulator to be fed back to the surgeon.

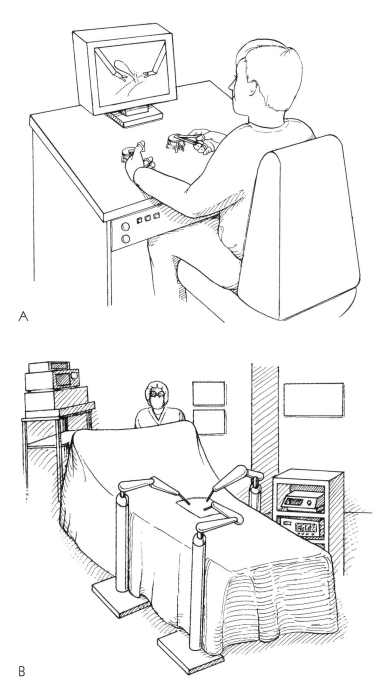

Fig. 10-2. Teleoperative surgery. **(A)** Motions of the controller handles operated by the surgeon are **(B)** transmitted to slave manipulators inside the patient. The handles exert forces on the surgeon's hands proportional to the forces resulting from manipulator contact with tissue.

These are most accurately measured at the instrument tip. Consequently, small sensors must be developed to gauge these forces.

The master controller should have a handle that the surgeon can grasp, perhaps shaped like the handle of a conventional surgical instrument. The device must be able to move in six dimensions and exert forces on the user's hand proportional to the forces sensed in contact between the slave manipulator and tissue. Master controller input could be scaled to control slave devices of different sizes, including microsurgical manipulators.[51] The major difficulty in designing a master controller is that it must have low mass and friction compared with the forces exerted by the surgeon. It is difficult to design a rigid mechanism with six actuators that is not massive and does not have friction in the force transmission mechanisms.[52]

Another major loss in laparoscopic surgery is the ability to palpate tissue. The human finger can sense a wide range of tissue properties such as surface shape and texture, mass, hardness, pulsation, and slip.[53] The design of devices to detect and display these features is an active but young area of teleoperation research. Fortunately, some of the tactile mechanisms most important to the surgeon, such as detecting the pulse of an artery hidden in fat, may be relatively easy to duplicate.[54] The most useful tactile aids will mount onto existing laparoscopic instruments. Consequently, tactile technology can develop independent of the master-slave telemanipulation devices described above.

Although technology such as this may seem too expensive and complex, it is rapidly evolving. The potential of medical applications will serve as an impetus for teleoperation research and for conversion of existing technology to surgical uses. Technology will probably be applied initially to applications where the needs are greatest: remote surgery, especially for military applications; microsurgical applications at the limits of human abilities; and hazardous applications where exposure to radioactive sources or highly transmissible diseases is a concern. As technology develops, it may become economical enough to be used more widely.

In other laparoscopic applications, robotics technology may be useful. Robots have already been used for their accuracy in stereotactic neurosurgery,[55,56] preparation of the femoral canal for total hip replacement,[57] and prostate resection.[58] In each case, imaging data from computed tomography, magnetic resonance imaging, or ultrasound are used to supply precise three-dimensional data. Unfortunately, abdominal organs are soft and mobile, so it will be difficult to transfer this technology directly to laparoscopic surgery.

Another application for robots is as surgical assistants.[47] Commercial robotic systems already exist to control laparoscope positioning.[59] It remains to be seen, however, if robotic assistants can overcome the economic limitations that have constrained the widespread use of industrial robots. It is difficult for a robot designed for a single application to be more economical than a human assistant. While the robot may be more efficient at one job, the versatility of a human worker often increases overall productivity.

Simulation for Training

As discussed in Chapter 9, learning laparoscopic surgery is very demanding. Although basic techniques can be learned in benchtop trainers, most procedures and skills currently must be taught in the animal laboratory. Differences between animal and human anatomy require that much must actually be learned in the process of operating on patients.

Computer technology is rapidly evolving to the point where realistic simulation of surgical anatomy will be possible. Just as airline pilots train on flight simulators, surgeons theoretically could train on surgical simulation devices. Such interactive simulations in which an environment is modeled so the user feels as if he or she is actually working in the simulated world are called *virtual environments* or *virtual reality*. Advantages of training with a surgical simulator would include accurate human anatomy, realistic interaction, and the ability to practice a technique or procedure repeatedly until skills are perfected.

Surgical simulation requires a computer capable of modeling tissue mechanics and graphically displaying tissue behavior. Simulator input devices must feel like laparoscopic instruments to provide realistic interaction. Unlike common computer joysticks, the devices must be capable of exerting forces on the surgeon's hand in proportion to the simulated tissue reaction forces.

The major technical difficulty in creating realistic simulation of the surgical environment is the large amount of computer power necessary.[60] To model and display the shapes of internal anatomy, surfaces and volumes must be mathematically broken up into elements. Many elements are necessary for realistic modeling of complex anatomic shapes. The simulation must model not only the surface appearance of tissue, but the mechanical properties as well. Furthermore, calculations for each of the elements must be performed at least 15 to 30 times a second, the rate at which simulated motion appears reasonably smooth to the user.[61] Computer workstations exist with hardware optimized to quickly perform perspective and lighting calculations for graphic rendering. More work must be done, however, in developing software algorithms and hardware architectures to model tissue mechanical behavior realistically. As computer power increases and prices drop, it is likely that simulation will become practical for surgical training.

References

1. Mouiel J, Katkhouda N: Laparoscopic vagotomy for chronic duodenal ulcer disease. World J Surg 17:34, 1993
2. Dubois F: Laparoscopic vagotomies. p. 348. In Berci G, Cuscheri A, Sackier JM (eds): Problems in General Surgery: Laparoscopic Surgery. JB Lippincott, Philadelphia, 1991
3. Graham DY, Lew GM, Klein PD et al: Effect of treatment of Helicobacter pylori infection on the long-term recurrence of gastric and duodenal ulcer. A randomized, controlled study [see comments]. Ann Intern Med 116:705, 1992
4. Hosking SW, Ling TK, Chung SC et al: Duodenal ulcer healing by eracidation of Helicobacter pylori without anti-acid treatment: randomised controlled trial. Lancet, 343:508, 1994
5. Nagai H, Kondo Y, Yasuda T et al: An abdominal wall-lift method of laparoscopic cholecystectomy without peritoneal insufflation. Surg Laparosc Endosc 3:175, 1993
6. Smith RS, Fry WR, Tsoi EK et al: Gasless laparoscopy and conventional instruments. The next phase of minimally invasive surgery. Arch Surg 128:1102, 1993
7. Newman L III, Luke JP, Ruben DML et al: Laparoscopic herniorrhaphy without pneumoperitoneum. Surg Laparosc Endosc 3:213, 1993
8. Hill D, Maher P, Wood C et al: Gasless laparoscopy. Aust N Z J Obstet Gynaecol 34:79, 1994
9. McKernan JB, Laws HL: Laparoscopic Nissen fundoplication for the treatment of gastroesophageal reflux disease. Am Surg 60:87, 1994
10. Kerbl K, Figenshau RS, Clayman RV et al: Retroperitoneal laparoscopic nephrectomy: laboratory and clinical experience. J Endourol 7:23, 1993
11. Gaur DD, Agarwal DK, Khochikar MV et al: Laparoscopic renal biopsy via retroperitoneal approach. J Urol 151:925, 1994
12. Rassweiler JJ, Henkel TO, Potempa DM et al: The technique of transperitoneal laparoscopic nephrectomy, adrenalectomy and nephroureterectomy. Eur Urol 23:425, 1993

13. Webb DR, Redgrave N, Chan Y et al: Extraperitoneal laparoscopy: early experience and evaluation. Aust N Z J Surg 63:554, 1993

14. Rassweiler JJ, Henkel TO, Stoch C et al: Retroperitoneal laparoscopic nephrectomy and other procedures in the upper retroperitoneum using a balloon dissection technique. Eur Urol 25:229, 1994

15. Childers JM, Hatch KD, Tran AN, Surwit EA: Laparoscopic para-aortic lymphadenectomy in gynecologic malignancies. Obstet Gynecol 82:741, 1993

16. Querleu D, LeBlanc E: Laparoscopic infrarenal paraaortic lymph node dissection for restaging of carcinoma of the ovary or fallopian tube. Cancer 73:1467, 1994

17. Dion YM, Katkhouda N, Rouleau C et al: Laparoscopy-assisted aorto-bifemoral bypass. Surg Laparosc Endosc 3:425, 1993

18. Poppas D, Sutaria P, Sosa RE et al: Chromophore enhanced laser welding of canine ureters in vitro using a human protein solder: a preliminary step for laparoscopic tissue welding. J Urol 150:1052, 1993

19. Pellegrini C, Wetter LA, Patti M et al: Thoracoscopic esophagomyotomy. Initial experience with a new approach for the treatment of achalasia. Ann Surg 216:291, 1992

20. Shimi SM, Nathanson LK, Cuschieri A: Thoracoscopic long oesophageal myotomy for nutcracker oesophagus: initial experience of a new surgical approach. Br J Surg 79:533, 1992

21. Gossot D, Forquier P, Celerier M: Thoracoscopic esophagectomy: technique and initial results. Ann Thorac Surg 56:667, 1993

22. Gossot D, Ghnassia MD, Debiolles H et al: Thoracoscopic dissection of the esophagus: an experimental study. Surg Endosc 6:59, 1992

23. Miller DL, McManus KG, Allen MS et al: Results of surgical resection in patients with N2 non-small cell lung cancer. Ann Thorac Surg 57:1095, 1994

24. Landreneau RJ, Dowling RD, Castillo WM et al: Thoracoscopic resection of an anterior mediastinal tumor [see comments]. Ann Thorac Surg 54:142, 1992

25. Rendina EA, Venuta F, De Giacomo T et al: Comparative merits of thoracoscopy, mediastinoscopy, and mediastinotomy for mediastinal biopsy. Ann Thorac Surg 57:992, 1994

26. Elia S, Cecere C, Giampaglia F et al: Mediastinoscopy vs. anterior mediastinotomy in the diagnosis of mediastinal lymphoma: a randomized trial. Eur J Cardiothorac Surg 6:361, 1992

27. Burke RP, Chang AC: Video-assisted thoracoscopic division of a vascular ring in an infant: a new operative technique. J Cardiac Surg 8:537, 1993

28. Lavoie J, Burrows FA, Gentles TL et al: Transoesophageal echocardiography detects residual ductal flow during video-assisted thoracoscopic patent ductus arteriosus interruption. Can J Anaesth 41:310, 1994

29. Buess G, Becker HD: Minimally invasive surgery in tumors of the esophagus. Langenbecks Archiv Chir, suppl 2:1355, 1990

30. Forster R: Thoracoscopic clipping of patent ductus arteriosus in premature infants. Ann Thorac Surg 56:1418, 1993

31. Maehara T, Ohgami M, Kokaji K et al: An innovative thoracoscopic surgery for patient ductus arteriosus—a Japanese first case report. J Jpn Assoc Thoracic Surg 41:1522, 1993

32. Way LW, Mori T, Legha P: Laparoscopic pancreatic cystgastrostomy: the first operation in the new field of intraluminal laparoscopic surgery. Arch Surg, in press

33. Ohashi S: Laparoscopic intra-gastric surgery: is it a new concept in lap surgery? Presented at the SAGES meeting, Nashville, TN, 1994

34. Ohgami M, Watanabe M, Kumai K et al: Laparoscopic curative wedge resection for the early gastric and early colon cancer using a lesion lifting method. Presented at the SAGES meeting, Nashville, TN, 1994

35. Harrison MR, Adzick NS: The fetus as a patient: surgical considerations. Ann Surg 213:279, 1991

36. Longaker MT, Golbus MS, Filly RA, et al: Maternal outcome after open fetal surgery. A review of the first 17 cases. JAMA 265:737, 1991

37. Harrison MR, Bressack MA, Churg AM et al: Correction of congenital diaphragmatic hernia in utero. II. Simulated correction permits fetal lung growth with survival at birth. Surgery 88:260, 1980

38. Natori M, Tanaka M, Kohno H et al: A case of twin–twin transfusion syndrome treated with placental vessel occlusion using fetoscopic Nd:YAG laser system. Acta Obstet Gynaecol Jpn 44(1):117, 1992

39. De Lia JE, Cruikshank DP, Keye WR, Jr: Fetoscopic neodymium:YAG laser occlusion of placental vessels in severe twin–twin transfusion syndrome. Obstet Gynecol 75:1046, 1990

40. Estes JM, Whitby DJ, Lorenz HP et al: Endoscopic creation and repair of fetal cleft lip. Plast Reconstr Surg 90:750, 1992

41. Tendick F, Jennings RW, Tharp G et al: Sensing and manipulation problems in endoscopic surgery: experiment, analysis, and observation. Presence 2:66, 1993

42. Cole RE, Merritt JO, Fore S, Lester P: Remote manipulator tasks impossible without stereo TV. p. 255. In Merritt JO, Fisher SS (eds): Stereoscopic Displays and Applications. Vol 1256. SPIE, Bellingham, WA, 1990

43. Mitchell TN, Robertson J, Nagy AG et al: Three-dimensional endoscopic imaging for minimal access surgery. J R Coll Surg Edinb 38:285, 1993

44. Diner DB, Fender DH: Human Engineering in Stereoscopic Viewing Devices. Plenum, New York, 1993

45. Pichler CV, Radermacher K, Grablowitz V et al: An ergonomic analysis of stereo-video-endoscopy. p. 1408. In Szeto AYJ, Rangayyan RM (eds): Proceedings of the IEEE Engineering in Medicine and Biology Society 15th Annual International Conference. IEEE, Piscataway, NJ, 1993

46. Sheridan TB: Telerobotics, Automation, and Human Supervisory Control. MIT Press, Cambridge, MA, 1992

47. Funda J, Taylor R, Eldridge B et al: Image-guided command and control of a surgical robot. p. 52. In: Medicine Meets Virtual Reality II: Interactive Technology & Healthcare: Visionary Applications for Simulation Visualization Robotics. Aligned Management Associates, San Diego, CA, 1994

48. Cohn MB, Crawford LS, Wendlandt JM, Sastry SS: Millirobotics for telesurgery. In: Proceedings of the First International Symposium on Medical Robotics and Computer Assisted Surgery. Pittsburgh, PA, 1994

49. Hollerbach JM, Hunter IW, Ballantyne J: A Comparative analysis of actuator technologies for robotics. p. 299. In Khatib O, Craig JJ, Lozano-Perez T (eds): Robotics Review 2. MIT Press, Cambridge, MA, 1991

50. Cain P, Kazanzides P, Zuhars J: Safety considerations in a surgical robot. Biomed Sci Instrum 29:291, 1993

51. Charles S, Williams RE, Hamel B: Design of a surgeon–machine interface for teleoperated microsurgery. p. 883. In Kim Y, Spelman FA (eds): Proceedings of the IEEE Engineering in Medicine and Biology Society 11th Annual International Conference. IEEE, New York, 1989

52. Millman PA, Stanley M, Colgate JE: Design of a high performance haptic interface to virtual environments. p. 216. In: Proceedings, IEEE Virtual Reality International Symposium. IEEE, Piscataway, NJ, 1993

53. Shimoga K: A survey of perceptual feedback issues in dexterous telemanipulation. Part II. Finger touch feedback. p. 263. In: Proceedings, IEEE Virtual Reality International Symposium. IEEE, Piscataway, NJ, 1993

54. Peine WJ, Son JS, Howe RD: A palpation system for artery localization in laparoscopic surgery. In: Proceedings of the First International Symposium on Medical Robotics and Computer Assisted Surgery. Pittsburgh, PA, 1994

55. Kwoh YS, Hou J, Jonckheere E, Hayati S: A robot with improved absolute positioning accuracy for CT guided stereotactic brain surgery. IEEE Trans Biomed Eng 35:153, 1988

56. Lavallee S, Troccaz J, Gaborit L et al: Image guided operating robot: a clinical application in stereotactic neurosurgery. p. 618. In: Proceedings 1992 IEEE

International Conference on Robotics and Automation. IEEE Computing Society Press, Los Alamitos, CA, 1992

57. Taylor RH, Mittelstadt BD, Paul HA et al: An image-directed robotic system for precise orthopaedic surgery. IEEE Trans Robotics Auto 10:261, 1994

58. Ng WS, Davies BL, Hibberd RD, Timoney AG: Robotic surgery. IEEE Eng Med Biol 12:120, 1993

59. Anonymous: Mission accomplished. NASA Tech Briefs 18:16, 1994

60. Satava RM: Virtual reality surgical simulator. The first steps. Surg Endosc 7:203, 1993

61. Liu A, Tharp G, French L et al: Some of what one needs to know about using head-mounted displays to improve teleoperator performance. IEEE Trans Robotics Auto 9:638, 1993

Index

Page numbers followed by *f* indicate figures; those followed by *t* indicate tables.

A

Abdomen
  cavity, inspection of, 128
  distension, 24–25, 89
    asymmetric, 170, 203
    bradycardia and, 202
    symmetrical, 94
  exiting, 128f–131f, 128–132
  incisions, multiple prior, 170t, 171
  lifting devices, 205, 236
  muscle relaxation
    anesthetic technique and, 187
    insufficient, 173
  pain, in right lower quadrant, 6
  wall
    bleeding, 208
    heavy, pneumoperitoneum estab-
      lishment and, 170, 170t
    retraction systems, 32–34, 34f
    tension, increasing, 95
Aberdeen knot, 142, 151, 152f
Accommodation, visual, 241
Acidosis, metabolic, 201
Active electrode, 57
Adhesions, postoperative intra-abdomi-
  nal, 4, 214–215
Adrenalectomy, open, 174–175
Air insufflator. *See* Insufflator
Airway management, 188

Alice forceps, 41, 98
Allen type low lithotomy stirrups, 162,
  163f
Alveolar-arterial oxygen gradient, 189
Analgesia, postoperative, 196–197
Anastomosis
  aortic, 237
  bowel, 114, 115f, 127
  intestinal, 49, 50
Anastomosis devices, 35. *See also* Linear
  cutter(s)
Anesthesia
  goals for intraoperative care, 187
  historical perspectives, 185
  induction, hemodynamic effects,
    188–189
  intraoperative
    monitoring, 191, 193–194
    physiologic changes/complications,
      188t, 188–191
  plan, 187–188, 192t–193t, 194
  postanesthesia care, 197
  preoperative considerations, 186–187
  techniques, 194–196
  type, 187
Anesthetic agents, 194
Animal training courses
  advantages, 228–229
  costs, 229
  methods/limitations, 230

Anterior abdominal wall retraction systems, 32–34, 34f
Anticholinesterase agents, 195
Antifogging solutions, 17, 157
Antireflux procedures
    complications, 200t, 216–218
    pig as surgical model for, 229
Antithromboembolic stockings, 166
Anvil, low-profile, 50, 51, 51f
Aorta puncture, accidental, 206
Aortobifemoral bypass, 237
Aortoiliac vascular disease, 237
Appendectomy
    clinical trials, 235–236
    complications, 200t, 215
    countertraction, 86
    history of, 7–8
    incidence, 6
    patient positioning, 86, 174
    Roeder loop usage, 107, 108f
Appendix
    retrieval, 125, 126
    rupture, 215
    stump fistula, 215
Argon-enhanced electrosurgery, 63–64
Argon laser, 65t
Arterial carbon dioxide tension, 190, 190t
Arthroscopy, 1
Aspirator use, proper, 117
Assistants, surgical, 5
    location, 81, 83
    robotic, 243
    role, 81, 85
Assisting ports, 89, 91f, 92, 97
Assisting trocars, insertion, 97–98
Atracurium, 195
Axis of operation, 81, 81f

B

Babcock clamp, 34, 37f, 41, 86, 120, 209
Ball electrodes, 118
Bilary tree surgery, patient positioning, 86

Bile, aspirated, retrieval, 125
Bile duct injury
    classification, 210, 211f
    clinical manifestations, 212
    postcholecystectomy, 210f, 210–213
    repair, 212
Bile duct stones, ultrasound diagnosis, 69
Biliary fistula, 213
Biliary operations, patient positioning, 174
Biliary stricture formation, 118
Bilirubin, 64
Binocular disparity, 240
Biopsy, laparoscopic, 2
Bipolar electrocautery. *See* Electrosurgery, bipolar systems
Bladder injuries, 207, 215
Bleeding. *See* Hemorrhage
Blind technique. *See* Closed technique
Blood pressure, intraoperative monitoring, 193
Blood vessel dissection, 121–122, 123f, 124
Bookwalter retractor, 158
Bowel
    anastomosis, 114, 115f, 127, 225
    injuries, 209
    perforation, 207
        risk factors, 207
        with Veress needle, 203
    prior distension, 170, 170t
    suturing, 4
Bowel clamp, 42
Brachial plexus injuries, 205
Bradycardia, 202
Bronchial carcinoma, thorascopic procedures, 73
Bruening's electroscope, 2

C

Calot's triangle, 70
    in animals, 229

en face view, 16
exposure, 212
retraction, 174
Camera operator
angled scopes and, 90
location, 81, 83
role, 83, 85
Camera system
cables, defective, 179
checking, 177–178
color balance, 176t, 179
console box, preoperative check, 165
declination, 83
design features, 18
focus, 176t, 179
gain, 19
head, checking for damage, 177
image quality, 85
iris, 19
one-chip, 18
resolution of, 18
panoramic view, 85
resolution of, 18–19
second camera, 21
separate, 17–18
signal
digital processing of, 20–21
types of, 18, 20
silicon chip. See Charge-coupling device
(CCD)
sterilization, 21–22
three-chip, 18, 139
tight or zoom view, 85
white balance, 19
Cannula(s), 29, 238. See also Trocar-cannula apparatus
additional, insertion of, 97–98
for assisting instruments, 91f, 92
diameter, 32
direct coupling of electrosurgical current and, 59–60, 60f
disposable, 29, 30f
flap valve, 100–101
gaining access to operative space and,
89

Hasson, 98
for operating instruments, 90, 91f, 92
O-ring, 30f, 31–32
reducer valve, 31–32
removal, 129
reusable, 29, 31f, 32, 96
self-retaining collar (fascial thread),
94–95, 157
site. See Ports
sleeves, capacitive coupling and, 61
standard, disadvantage of Hasson technique, 98
for thoracic surgery, 74
valves, 30, 30f, 31f
Capacitive coupling, of electrosurgical
current and, 60–61
Capacitors, 60–61
Caput medusa, 208
Carbon dioxide
end-tidal, 190, 190t, 191, 193
insufficient at source, 171t, 172
insufflation, 89, 187, 207
advantages of, 201
in closed technique, 92–93
leakage from system, 171t, 173
medical grade, 25
metabolic effects, 201
obstructed flow, 171t, 172f, 172–173
peritoneal absorption, 201
pneumothorax, 202
Carbon dioxide embolism, 94, 170, 201,
203
Carbon dioxide laser, 65, 65t
Carbonization, 63
Cardiac arrest, Veress needle malposition
and, 170
Cardiopulmonary bypass, for carbon
dioxide embolism, 203
Cardiovascular collapse, during laparoscopic surgery, 203, 204
Cardiovascular disease, 201
Castroviejo handle, 36f, 39
Cathode ray tube (CRT), 241
Cautery unit, 158, 159

Cavitating devices, ultrasonic, 71
Cavitation, 70
CCD. *See* Charge-coupling device (CCD)
Central venous pressure (CVP), 193
Charge-coupling device (CCD)
  defined, 18
  electronic iris and, 19
  signal
    digital processing of, 20
    types of, 20
  vision enhancement and, 240
Chemical sterilization, of camera unit,
    21–22
Cholecystectomy
  acceptance of, 1
  anesthesia morbidity, 185
  animal training course, 230
  Calot's triangle, en face view of, 16
  complications, 200t
    bile duct injury, 210f, 210–213
    biliary fistula without common duct
      injury, 213
    gallstone spillage, 214
    hemorrhage, 213
  criteria, 6–7
  first, 1, 6
  history of, 6–7
  operative site, 89
  outpatient, 187
  patient criteria, 6–7
  postanesthesia care, 197
  traction and countertraction, 86, 88f
  training, 7, 225–226
  ventilatory parameters, 189–191, 190t
Choledocoscopy, 17
Cholelithiasis, 186
Chromophores, 64
Chronic obstructive pulmonary disease
    (COPD), 186
Chylothorax, thoracoscopic procedures, 73
Circular staplers, 48, 50–51, 51f
  use, proper, 114, 116f, 116–117
Circumferential window, for blood vessel
    dissection, 122, 123f, 124

Cirrhosis, laparoscopic identification, 2
Clip appliers, 4, 74, 238
  features, important, 46–47, 47f
  half-way squeezed clip technique
    (teardrop), 124
  materials, choice of, 46–47
  sizes, 46
  teardrop shape, 109, 110f
  titanium, 46
  use, proper, 107, 109, 110f
Clips, mechanical
  dislodgement, 209–210
  inappropriate placement, 209–210
Closed technique, 89
  conversion
    to laparotomy, 93
    to open technique, 182
  disadvantages, 98
  insertion of Veress needle, 92–93
  trocar insertion, 94–98, 96f
    insertion of additional cannulas,
      97–98
  Veress needle for, 27–28, 28f
Coagulation, 57
Coagulation tests, 186
Coaxial handles, 36f, 37, 39, 140
Coaxial set-up, 81, 81f, 83
Coin lesions, thoracoscopic procedures,
    73
Cold light source, 3, 23
Colectomy, 54, 117, 236
  complications, 200t, 216
  operative site, 89
  port placement, 92
Colon
  mobilization, laparoscopic, 86
  prior distension, 170, 170t
  specimen retrieval, 125
Colon resection
  angled scopes for, 90
  assistant surgeon role, 81
  with colostomy, tissue removal tech-
    nique, 125
  partial, T-fastener usage, 106

Colorectal surgery, laparoscopic, 34
Common bile duct exploration, 21
Common hepatic duct, involvement in
        cystic duct clip, 107
Composite video signal, 20, 23
Compression stockings, 166
Computed tomography (CT), 5, 212
Computer simulation, for training,
        230–231, 247–248
Condom, as tissue retrieval device, 54, 126
Continuous documentation recording, 24
Continuous suture, 142, 151, 152f
Convergence, 241
Cooper scissors, 42
Cooper's ligament, 109, 214
COPD (chronic obstructive pulmonary
        disease), 186
Coronary artery disease, 186
Cost
    animal training courses, 229
    disposable and reusable instruments,
        35–36
    laparoscopic procedures, 35–36
Countertraction, 85, 86, 88f–89f, 174
Cricoid pressure, 194
Crochet knot (Aberdeen knot), 151, 152f
Crosstalk, 241
CRT (cathode ray tube), 241
CT (computed tomography), 5, 212
Culdoscopy, 3
Curare, 195
Cutting instruments. See also Scissors;
        Trocar(s)
    disposable, 35
    ultrasonic, 71, 159
Cystic duct occlusion, clip applier for, 107
Cystoscope, 2
Cystoscopy, 1

D

Debulking, 126
Deep venous thrombosis, 94, 203–204

Defogging solution, 178
Degrees of freedom, 242–243, 243f
Dejardin forceps, 55
Delivery apparatus, 27
Delivery pressure, gas flow rate and, 27
Desiccation, tissue, 57
Dexterity enhancement, for laparoscopic
        surgery, 239, 242–244, 243f, 245f,
        246–247
Diaphragm displacement, by pneu-
        moperitoneum, 201–202
Differential lung ventilation, 237
Digital contrast enhancement, 241–242
Digital signal processing, 20–21
Direct coupling, of electrosurgical cur-
        rent, 59–60, 60f
Disposable instruments. See also specific
        instruments
    advantages, 35
    disadvantages, 35–36
    vs. reusable instruments, 35–36, 36f
Dissection
    blood vessels, 121–122, 123f, 124
    soft tissue, 120–121, 122f
    ultrasonic, 71
Dissector(s), 38f, 39
    blunt dissection technique, 121, 122f
    design features, 40–41
    injuries, accidental, 102, 102f
    jaws, 101
    limited tactile feedback of, 40
    plucking, 122f
    raking, 122f
    as rod-like retractors, 101
    rotation of jaws, 42
    size, 41
    surface of jaws, 41–42
    tactile feedback, 101
    ultrasonic, 121–122
    ultrasound, tissue selectivity of, 70, 71f
    use, proper, 101–103, 102f
Distal closure, 46
Distortion, signal, 20–21
Dormia basket, 214

Dot pitch, 22–23
Double-action movement instruments, 42
Doxacurium, 195
Droperidol, 197
Drop test, 93
Dual trocar technique, 2
Duodenum injuries, 215
Dysphagia, postoperative, 217

E

ECGs (electrocardiograms), 186
Ectopic pregnancies, laparoscopic man-
    agement of, 4
Elderly, 25, 186
Electrical interference, video imaging and,
    180
Electricity, tissue effects, 57, 58f–59f
Electrocardiograms (ECGs), 186
Electrocautery. *See* Electrosurgery
Electrodes
  active, 56
  ball, 118
  hook, 118, 119f
  point, 118
  return or dispersive, 56
  spatula, 118, 119f
  tip designs, 61–62, 62f
Electrosurgery, 55–56, 75
  argon-enhanced, 63–64
  bipolar systems
    design features, 57, 62–63, 63f
    scissors, 120
    use, proper, 119–120
  electrical interference from, 180
  hazards, 57, 59–61
    capacitive coupling, 60–61
    direct coupling, 59–60, 60f
    insulation break, 59
  for hemostasis, 129–130
  injuries, 209
    alternate site burn, 56
    ground reference systems and, 61

  isolation burn, 61
    pad site burn, 56
  instruments, insulation on, 181
  monopolar systems, 56
    coagulation, 57
    design features, 56–57, 61–62, 62f
    electrode tip design, 61–62, 62f
    foot switch, 61
    handsets, 61
    rocker switch, 61
    use, proper, 117–118
    wave forms, 58f
  scissors, 103
  tissue effects electricity and, 57, 58f–59f
Emphysema
  bullous, 73
  subcutaneous, 54, 203
Empyema drainage, 8
Endometrial implant coagulation, 4
Endometriomas, 66
Endoscope, development, 1–2
Endoscopic retrograde cholangiopancre-
    atography (ERCP), 212
Endoscopic surgery
  history, 1
  laser applications, 66–67
Endotracheal intubation, 188
End-tidal carbon dioxide, 190, 190t, 193
Enterostomy, T-fastener usage, 106
Enterotomy, 127, 207, 238
Epidural analgesia, 197
Epidural anesthesia, 187
Equipment. *See also specific types of equip-
    ment*
  operating room, 156, 157–158
  preoperative check, 164–166
ERCP (endoscopic retrograde cholan-
    giopancreatography), 212
Eschar formation, 63
Esophageal motor disorders, 237
Esophageal perforation, spontaneous, 8
Esophageal reflux, 186
Esophageal stethoscope, 194
Esophagectomy, 237

Esophagus, abdominal, operations on, 86
Ethylene oxide sterilization, of camera unit, 21
Exposure
    gasless laparoscopy and, 236–237
    intraluminal access, 238–239
    mediastinal, 237–238
    methods, 24–27, 26f, 85
    problems in, 173–175, 174t
    retroperitoneal, 237
Extracorporeal knotting, 151, 153, 153f
Extracorporeal shockwave lithotripsy, 6
Extraperitoneal insufflation, 203

F

Fallopian tube
    direct microsurgical repair of, 4
    occlusion, clip applier for, 107
Fan retractors, 74
    features, important, 43–44, 44f
    use, proper, 104, 105f
Fascial threads (self-retaining collar), 94–95, 157
Femoral nerve mononeuropathies, 205
Fetoscopic surgery, 239
Fever, postoperative, 215
Fiber-optic light cord, 157
Fiber-optic scopes
    advantages, 17
    bundle damage, 23
    field of view, 17
    for thoracoscopic surgery, 73–74
Fluid therapy, intravenous, 195
Fluoroscopy operating room set-up, supine, 159–160, 161f, 162f
Foley catheter insertion, for bleeding control, 129, 129f, 208
Forward viewing scope, 16
French knot (Aberdeen knot), 151, 152f
Frimbiolysis, 4
Fulguration, 57

G

Gain, camera, 19–20
Galactomer suture material, 141
Gallbladder
    fixed retraction, 81
    perforation, 214
    specimen retrieval, 126
    tumors, ultrasound diagnosis, 69
Gallstones, 186
    dissolution therapy, 6
    intraperitoneal, 214
    retrieval, 125
    spillage, in cholecystectomy, 213
Gas(es)
    carbon dioxide See Carbon dioxide
    choice of, 25
    flow rate
        delivery pressure and, 26–27
        impedance and, 27
        insufflator and, 25–27
        maximal, 27
    helium, 25, 204
    nitrous oxide, 25, 204
    for pneumoperitoneum establishment, 204
    warming of, 25
Gas bloat, postoperative, 217
Gas embolism, 203. See also Carbon dioxide embolism
Gas sterilization, of camera unit, 21
Gastrectomy, 229
Gastric emptying, 186, 194
Gastric operations, patient positioning, 174
Gastric resection, partial, T-fastener usage, 106
Gastroesophageal junction, surgical set-up, 83
Gastroesophageal reflux, symptomatic, 194
Gastrointestinal anastomosis device. See Linear cutter(s)
Gastrointestinal tract, upper surgery, patient positioning, 86
Gastrojejunostomy, 114, 115f, 229

Gastroscopy device, 2
Ghosting, 180
GIA devices (gastrointestinal anastomosis
    devices), 47, 49f, 49–50
Glare, 180
Glassman clamps, 41, 120
Glutaraldehyde sterilization, of camera
    unit, 21–22
Granny knot, 143
Grasper(s), 74
    assisting ports, 91f, 92
    atraumatic, 41–42
    design features, 37f, 39, 41
    injuries, accidental, 102, 102f, 209
    jaws, 41–42, 101, 140
    limited tactile feedback of, 40
    to pull organ in opposite directions,
        86–87, 89f
    as rod-like retractors, 101
    rotation of jaws, 42
    size, 41
    in suturing, 140
    tactile feedback, 101
    tip-to-tip approximation method and,
        111, 112f
    tissue retrieval technique, 125
    training, 142–143
    use, proper, 101–103, 102f, 140
    X approximation method and, 111, 112f
Gravity countertraction, 85, 86, 88f
Ground reference systems, 56

H

Half circle needles, 142
Hand-eye coordination, visual perception
    and, 139–140
Handle(s)
    Castroviejo, 36f, 39
    circular stapler, 50, 51f
    clip applier, 46, 47f
    hernia stapler, 48
    linear cutter, 49, 49f

linear or coaxial, 36f, 37, 39, 140
    operating instruments, 36f, 37, 39
    Roman scissors, 36f, 37, 80, 140
Hasson cannula, 32, 33f, 98
Hasson technique. See Open technique
Heart disease, 186
Heart murmur, in carbon dioxide embo-
    lism, 203
Helicobacter pylori infection, 235
Helium, 25, 204
Heller cardiomyotomy, 229
Hemoglobin, 64, 186
Hemorrhage, 180
    abdominal wall, 208
    in cholecystectomy, 213
    control, 57, 124, 180–181
        bipolar energy for, 62
        clip applier for, 109
        electrocautery for, 129–130
        Foley catheter insertion for, 129,
            129f
        through-and-through suture, 128f,
            129, 130
    intra-abdominal, 191
    intra-abdominal pressure and, 128
    postoperative, 215
    prevention, 124
Hemothorax, 73
Hepatic lesions, ultrasound diagnosis,
    69
Hernia, paraesophageal, 217
Hernia staplers, 47
    design features, 48f, 48–49
    inappropriate usage, 127
    jaws, 111
    rotating device, 48f, 48–49
    tissue approximation methods
        partial staple deployment, 111, 113f
        tip-to-tip, 111, 112f
        X arrangement, 111, 112f
    use, proper, 109, 111, 112f
Herniation
    repair. See Herniorrhaphy
    trocar site, 208–209

Herniorrhaphy
clinical trials, 235–236
complications, 200t, 213–215
hernia recurrence rate and, 214–215
hernia stapler usage, 109, 111, 112f
inguinal, patient positioning, 174
operative site, 89
pig as surgical model for, 229–230
HIDA scan, of bile duct injury, 212
High-resolution monitor, 22–23
History
appendectomy, laparoscopic, 7–8
early clinical experience, 2
endoscope, 1–2
inception of laparoscopy, 2
laparoscopic cholecystectomy, 6–7
laparoscopy in general surgery, 5–6
technological advances and operative
techniques, 3–5
Hook electrodes, 118, 119f
Hook scissors, 103
Hopkins rod lens system, 13, 14f–15f, 23
Horizontal scan rate, 22
Hospital admission, 186
Hypercarbia, 201, 202
Hyperhidrosis, 73
Hypotension, 191, 203
Hypothermia prevention, 25

I

Ibuprofen, 196
Iliac artery puncture, 206
Iliac vein, flow disturbance, 94
Illumination
cold light source, 3
for endoscope, 2
insufficient, 178
problems, 177
Images, video
black spots in, 23–24
blurred, 176t, 179
dark grainy, 178

development/processing of, 24
digital contrast enhancement, 241–242
digitized, 24
with faded or inappropriate color, 176t,
179
foggy, 178–179
with glare/ghosting, 180
with interference lines, 180
jumpy, 179
obscured by blood, 124
poor-quality, 176t, 178–179
problems with, 175, 176t, 177f, 177–180
Imaging equipment. *See* Video imaging
equipment
Impedance, gas flow rate and, 27
Incisions
muscle-splitting gridiron, 125
Pfannenstiel, 125
vertical, 125
Induction agents, 194
Infection, at trocar site, 125
Informed consent, 156
Instruction, didactic, 226
Instrument holder, self-retaining, 52, 53f
Instruments. *See also specific instruments*
advances in, 13
assisting. *See also* Grasper(s); Retractor(s)
cannulas for, 91f, 92f
complications, 205–209
crossing. *See* Sword fighting
degrees of freedom, 242–243, 243f
extraction, 100–101
handle and shaft, 36f
imaging. *See* Video imaging equipment
insertion, 100
manual dexterity for, 80, 81f
mechanical failure, 180
new designs, 75
positioning, 174t, 175
retracting, 43–45, 44f–45f
self-retaining holder, 52, 53f
suturing, 140
tactile feedback, 80, 240
touch confirmation, 100

Insufflator(s)
  alarm system, 27
  automatic, 4
  carbon dioxide gas line, 99
  design features, 25, 26f
  gas, 89
  gas flow rate and, 25–27
  gas pressure, 27, 93–94
  high-flow, 26
  high pressure and low flow, 171t,
      172–173
  indicators, 27
  low pressure and high flow, 171t, 173
  low pressure and low flow, 171t, 172
  needle placement, gas pressure and,
      94
  preoperative check, 157–158, 159,
      165–166
  procedure
    extraperitoneal, 203
    incorrect, 203
  tubing, 17, 27, 157
Insulation break, of electrosurgical instru-
    ment, 59
Intercostal nerve blocks, 197
Intestinal anastomosis, 49, 50
Intra-abdominal abscess, 215
Intra-abdominal adhesions, after hernia
    repair, 215
Intra-abdominal pressure, 25–26
  bleeding and, 128
  elevations, hemodynamic effects, 202
  maintenance, 27
  monitoring of, 3–4
  in obese patients, 170
  rise, argon-enhanced electrosurgery
      and, 64
Intracorporeal anastomotic leak, 215
Intragastric surgery, 21
Intraluminal access, 238–239
Intraoperative monitoring, 191,
    193–194
In vitro training, 227–228
Iris, camera, 19

Irrigation fluid, 54, 117, 166
Irrigators, 4, 26, 117
Isolated systems, electrosurgical, 56–57

J

Jaws, instrument
  in blind insertion, 100
  clip applier, 46, 47f
  double-action, 42
  linear cutter, 49, 49f
  needle driver, 140
  operating instruments, 37f–38f, 39–40
  rotation feature, 42
  shape, 42–43
  single-action, 42
  size, 41
  surface, 41–42
Jejunostomy, 229

K

Keith needle, 132
Kelly clamp, 94, 129
Ketorolac, 196
Kidney, specimen retrieval, 125
Kinesthetic feedback, 239
Kinesthetic sensation, lack of, in operating
    instruments, 40
Kleppinger forceps, 120
Knotting, 137. See also specific knots
  extracorporeal, 151, 153, 153f
  intracorporeal, 143, 144f–149f, 150
Knot tying, intra- and extracorporeal, 4
Kocher clamps, 98
KTP laser, 65, 65t

L

Laboratory tests, preoperative, 186
Lactated Ringer's solution with heparin,
    117

Laparoscope(s)
    angulated, 15f, 16–17, 84f, 85, 90
    blinding, 17
    135 degree oblique view, 2
    design features, 13, 14f–15f, 16–17
    eyepiece fogging, 178–179
    field of view, 16
    5-mm, 16
    image. *See* Images, video
    insertion, 3
    limited viewing angle, 80
    positioning, 174t, 175
    rigid, 157
    scope, 16
    stereoscopic, 240–241
    sterilization, 179
    target area, 16
    10-mm, 16
    viewing angle, 84f, 85
    viewing lens obscured by blood, 180
    without angulation, 16
Laparoscope holder, 52, 53f, 83
Laparoscope warmer, 157
Laparoscopy, 132. *See also specific surgical
        procedures*
    acceptance of, 3
    clinical trials, 235
    coaxial set-up, 81, 81f
    complications
        of instrumentation, 205–209
        of patient position, 205
        predictors after training course, 232
    dexterity enhancement, 242–244, 243f,
        245f, 246–247
    early clinical experience, 2
    exposure, 236–239
    first experimental, 2
    future of, 8, 235–248
    gasless, 236–237
    in general surgery, 5–8
    inception of, 2
    limited perspective of, 16
    one-handed, 87
    operative techniques, advances in, 3–5

    perception enhancement, 239, 240–242
    privileging criteria, 231–232
    simulation for training, 247–248
    tactile feedback, 80
    technical complications, 199, 200t,
        201–205
    technical notes, 120–122, 122f, 123f, 124
    technological advances in, 3–5
    teleoperative, 244, 245f, 246–247
    terminology for, 2
    training. *See* Training
    two-handed, 87
    video-guided, 6
Laparotomy
    advantages, 125
    disadvantages, 125–126
Lasers, 55–56
    advantages, 5, 64–65
    contact systems, 66
    delivery, 65–66, 66f
    development, 64
    endoscopic surgery applications, 66–67
    history, 4–5
    injuries, 208
    medium, 65, 65t
    physics, 64–65
    pulsing, 66
    thoracoscopic surgery, 75
    vs. electrocautery, 7
Lasso knot, 150
Lateral decubitus position
    intra-abdominal pressure and, 170
    operating room set-up for, 163, 164f
Lens system, 16–17
Light source, 23–24, 178
Linea alba, 94
Linear cutter(s), 74
    bowel anastomosis, 127
    design features, 47, 49f, 49–50
    jaws, 111–114, 115f
    port sites, 113
    staple cartridges, 112
    staple depth, 111, 112
    use, proper, 113–114, 115f

Linear handles, 36f, 37, 39
Linear scanning ultrasound probes, 67,
    68f
Lithotomy position, nerve injuries during,
    205
Lithotripsy, 6
Liver function tests, 186
Liver injuries, 207–208, 209
Liver retractor, 120
Local anesthesia, 187
    for analgesic supplementation, 196
    without abdominal relaxation, 173
Low lithotomy, operating room set-up,
    162–163, 163f
Low-profile anvil, 50, 51, 51f
Lung disease, 186, 190–191, 191, 201
Lung resection, staple depth, 74
Lung retractors, 74, 86, 237
Lymph node sampling, mediastinal,
    237
Lymphomas, mediastinal, 73

M

Malignancy
    laparoscopic identification, 2
    seeding, at trocar site, 125
Master controller, 246
Materials, suture, 141
0-Maxon needle, 131
Mayo scissors, 42
Mechanical assistant. *See* Self-retaining
    arm
Median sternotomy, 203
Mediastinal access, 237–238
Mediastinal tumors, thorascopic proce-
    dures, 73
Mediastinoscopy, 237–238
Melanin, 64
Memory alloys, 244
Meperidine, 196, 197
Mesentery injuries, 207–208
Metabolic acidosis, 201

Methohexital, 194
Metzenbaum scissors, 42, 103
Microscissors, 42, 103
Midazolam, 194
Mill wheel murmur, in carbon dioxide
    embolism, 203
Minilaparotomy, 7, 54, 55, 125
Mirror image effect, 83
Misting, of objective lens, 17
Mivacurium, 195
Mobilization, laparoscopic, 86
Monitor(s), 139, 157
    accessory, 81
    compatibility with signal, 21
    ghost imaging, 23
    interfering images on, 179–180
    line input, video signal and, 177
    positioning, in operating room, 158–159
    preoperative check, 164–165
    scan rates, 22
    signal path to imaging equipment, 177,
        177f
    signal termination, 23
    surgeon location and, 81
    ultrasound, 69
Monofilament material, 141
Monopolar electrosurgical units. *See*
    Electrosurgery, monopolar systems
Morphine, 196, 197
Muscle relaxants, 187, 195

N

Naproxen, 196
National Television Standards Council
    (NTSC), 22
Nausea, postoperative, 197
Nd:YAG laser, 65, 65t, 66
Necrosis, tissue. *See* Desiccation, tissue
Needle(s). *See also specific needles*
    deflection, 142
    grasping point, 142
    insufflating (spring-loaded or Veress), 3

Needle driver, 140
Needle holders, 4, 34, 37
Nerve entrapment, after hernia repair,
    214
Nissen fundoplication, 92
Nitrous oxide, 25, 204
Nitze cystoscope, 2
Nonsteroidal anti-inflammatory agents,
    196
NTSC (National Television Standards
    Council), 22
Nylon tissue retrieval bag, 55

O

Obesity
    anesthetic implications, 186
    intra-abdominal pressure and, 170
    trocar insertion and, 95
    Veress needle length and, 170
Objective lens, temperature differences
    across, 17
Omental adhesions, 4
Ondansetron, 197
One-finger retractors, 44, 44f, 104, 105f
One-handed surgery, 87
One-lung ventilation, 196
Oophorectomy, 4
Open technique
    bowel perforation risk and, 207
    conversion to, 171, 182, 191
    history, 3
    instrumentation, 32, 33f, 98–99, 99f
    pneumoperitoneum creation, 32, 89
    procedure, 98–99, 99f
    removal of preperitoneal gas, 203
    skin incision, 93, 98
Operating field. *See* Operating space
Operating instruments, 35
    disposable *vs.* reusable, 35–36, 36f
    handles, 36f, 37, 39
    jaws, 37f–38f, 39–40
    limited tactile feedback of, 40

shaft, 39
typical, 36f–38f, 37, 39–43
Operating ports. *See* Ports, operating
Operating room
    laparoscopic equipment/supplies, 156,
        157
    set-up, 155, 156, 158–159
        lateral decubitus, 163, 164f
        low lithotomy, 162–163, 163f
        for pelvic procedures, 159, 161f
        supine, with fluoroscopy, 159–160,
            161f, 162f
        for upper abdominal and thoracic
            procedures, 159, 160f
        without fluoroscopy, 160, 162
    table, 158
    team, 155
Operating space
    characteristics, 79–80
    creating and maintaining, 24–27, 26f
    display, 85–87
    distance from ports, 90
    en face view, 16
    exposure. *See* Exposure
    gaining access, 89
    maintaining, in thorascopic surgery,
        74
    positioning of surgeon and, 80–81,
        81f–82f, 83
    unfamiliar view, 199
    video magnification, 80
    visual perception in, 79
Operative pelviscopy, 4
Opioids, 196
Ovarian mass, specimen retrieval, 125
Oxygen, supplemental, 197

P

PACU (postanesthesia care unit), 197
PAL standard, 22
Pancuronium, 195
Para-aortic lymph node dissection, 237

Paraesophageal hernia, 217
Patient
    position, 86
        complications, 205
        incorrect, 173–174, 174t
        right lateral decubitus, 86
        Trendelenburg. *See* Trendelenburg
            position
    preoperative check-in, 156
    surgical history, 156
PDS needle, 131
Pelvic procedures
    operating room set-up, 159, 161f
    patient position, 205
Pelvitrainer, 4
Penrose drains, 44, 107, 108f
Peptic ulcer disease, 48, 194
Pericardial effusion, malignant, thoras-
    copic procedures, 73
Peripheral nerve stimulator, 187–188, 195
Peritoneal cavity
    access. *See* Closed technique; Open
        technique
    gaseous distention. *See* Abdomen, dis-
        tension
Peritonitis, 213
Periumbilical varices, 208
Peroneal neuropathy, 205
Pfannenstiel incision, 125
pH, arterial, 201
Photon, 64
Piezoelectric crystals, 67, 69, 70
Pig, as surgical training model, 228–230
Pipecuronium, 195
Plastic molded instruments. *See* Dis-
    posable instruments
Plastic tissue retrieval bag, 54–55, 55f,
    126
Pleural effusions, 8, 73
Pleural thickening, 8
Pleural tumors, 73
Pneumoperitoneum
    alternatives, 204
    decompression, 191

establishment, 93–94. *See also* Operating
    space
    alternative gases, 204
    blind technique for, 25–26
    choice of gas for, 25
    by closed or blind technique. *See*
        Closed technique
    complications of, 200t, 201–204
    by open or Hasson technique. *See*
        Open technique
    problems in, 169–171, 170t
    hemodynamic effects, 202
    maintenance
        cannula removal and, 129
        problems in, 171t, 171–173, 172f
    pulmonary effects, 201
    venous tamponading effect, 128
Pneumoperitoneum needle, 3
Pneumo-preperitoneum, 170
Pneumothorax
    antireflux procedures and, 217
    carbon dioxide, 202
    tension, 202
    therapeutic thoracoscopy, 8
    thorascopic procedures, 73
Point electrodes, 118
Polarized filtering, 241
Polydiaxanone suture material, 141
Polyester suture material, 141
Polyglactin suture material, 141
Polypropylene suture material, 141
Polyurethane tissue retrieval bag, 54–55,
    55f, 126
Portal hypertension, 208
Ports, 89. *See also* Trocar(s); Trocar-can-
    nula apparatus
    assisting, 91f, 92
    bleeding, 128f–129f, 129
    closure, 130f, 131–132
    for instruments, 90, 91f, 92
    operating, 89, 90, 91f, 92
        angle between, 92
        closed technique, 97
        positioning, 174t, 175

scope, 89, 90, 97
siting, 89–90, 91f, 92, 113
tissue retrieval through, 54
triangulation of, 137–138, 138f
Positioning devices, 158
Postanesthesia care unit (PACU), 197
Prelooped suture, 150
Premedication, 194
Preoperative considerations, for anesthe-
   sia, 186
Preoperative equipment check, 164–166
Prochlormethazine, 197
Propofol, 194
Pseudoaneurysm, 209
Pseudocysts, pancreatic, 238–239
Pulmonary artery pressure, 193
Pulmonary capillary wedge pressure,
   193
Pulmonary embolism, 203–204
Pulse oximetry, 190
Pyloroplasty, 229

R

Radiography
   equipment, 158
   for retrieval of broken instrument parts,
      181
Recording equipment, 24
   compatibility with signal, 21
   continuous documentation procedure,
      24
   still picture recording, 24
Rectum, cul de sac, 125
Reducer valves, 100, 157
Refreshing rate, 22
Regional anesthesia, 173, 187
REM (return electrode monitoring), 56
Resolution, of one-chip camera, 18
Retraction, 86
   direction, 92
   forms of, 43
   inappropriate, 174t, 174–175

methods, 44–45, 45f, 107. *See also specific*
   retraction methods
of viscera, 85
Retractor(s), 74, 86
   assisting ports, 91f, 92
   basic requirements, 43
   design features, 43–45, 44f–45f
   features, important, 103
   injuries, 209
   solid organ, 43–44, 44f
   use, proper, 103–104, 105f, 106–107,
      108f
Retrieval, of broken instrument parts, 181
Retrieval bags, 125
Retroperitoneal access, 237
Retroperitoneal bleeding, 206
Return electrode monitoring (REM), 56
Reusable instruments. *See also specific*
   instruments
   advantages of, 35–36
RGB analog recorder, 24
RGB digital video recorder, 24
RGB signal, 20, 21, 23
Richter's hernia, 208
Right-angle retractors, 44, 86, 104, 105f
Right lateral decubitus position, 86
Rigid laparoscopes, 157
   design features, 13, 14f–15f, 16–17
   field of view, 16
   sizes, 16
Risk-to-benefit ratio, 199
Robotics technology, 244, 245f, 246–247
Rocuronium, 195
Rod lens system, 3, 13, 14f–15f, 139
Roeder knot, 151, 153f
Roeder loop, 4, 7
Roman scissors handles, 36f, 37, 140

S

SAGES (Society of American Gastrointestinal Endoscopic Surgeons), 231–232

Saline irrigation fluid, 117
Salpingolysis, 4
Salpingostomy, 4
Scissors, 38f, 39, 74
   angulated, 43, 103
   articulated, 103
   bipolar, 62–63, 63f, 120
   connectability to electrocautery unit, 43
   disposable, 42
   electrocautery, 103, 118–119
   injuries, accidental, 103
   monopolar, 62–63
   rotatability, 43
   shape of jaws, 42–43
   use, proper, 103
Scissors-type handles, 36f, 37
Scope cannula, insertion, 94–97, 96f
Scope ports, 89, 90, 97
Sector scanning ultrasound probes, 67
Sedative/hypnotic agents, 194
Self-retaining arm(s)
   design features, 51–52, 53f
   midchest level, 120
   use, proper, 120
Sequential compression stockings, 158
Set-up
   operating room. See Operating room,
      set-up
   procedural, 137–139, 138f
      coaxial, 137, 175
      triangulation of ports, 137–138, 138f
Shaft, operating instruments, 39
Sickle cell disease, 201
Signal. See Video signal
Signal-to-noise ratio, 18
Simulation, for training, 247–248
Single-action movement instruments,
   42
Single-surgeon technique, 87, 89
Ski needles, 141, 142
Skin incision
   closed laparoscopy, 93
   open laparoscopy (Hasson technique),
      98

Slave manipulators, 244, 245f
Slide makers, 24
Sliding knot, 151
Sling, 44, 107
Society for Surgeons of the Alimentary
      Tract (SSAT), 231–232
Society of American Gastrointestinal En-
      doscopic Surgeons (SAGES),
      231–232
Spatula electrodes, 118, 119f
Specimen removal, 124–126
Spinal anesthesia, 187
Spleen
   injuries, 207–208, 209
   specimen retrieval, 125, 126
Splenectomy, patient positioning, 86
Sponge forceps, 55
Sponge sticks, 34
Square knot, 142, 143, 144f–149f
SSAT (Society for Surgeons of the
      Alimentary Tract), 231–232
Staple
   depth
      after closure, 50
      for lung resection, 74
   dislodgement, 109
Staple cartridges, 49, 50
Stapling devices, 142. See also specific sta-
      pling devices
   advantages, for thoracoscopic surgery,
      74
   design features, 47–51, 48f, 49f
   disposable, 35
   tissue approximation, 126–127
   use, proper, 109, 111–114, 112f, 113f,
      115f, 116f, 116–117
Stereopsis, human, 240, 241
Sterile glove, for tissue retrieval, 54
Sterilization
   of camera unit, 21–22
   laparoscope, 179
   of laparoscopic instruments, 35
Steris system, 22, 179
Still picture recording, 24

Stomach
  operations, 86
  perforation, 207
Stopcock, for insufflating channel,
    95–96
Straight needles, 142
Succinylcholine, 195
Suction-irrigation devices, 52, 54, 62f, 74,
    157
Super-VHS image, 20
Surgeon(s)
  assistant. *See* Assistants, surgical
  left-handed, suture line for, 139
  location, 80–81, 82f–83f, 83
  position, 137
  right-handed, suture line for, 139
  training. *See* Training
Surgeon's knot, 142, 143, 144f–148f
Surgical glove, as retrieval device,
    126
Suture(s), 44
  cannula site closure, 130f, 131–132
  continuous, performing, 150–151,
    152f
  material, 141
  placement, in absence of pneumoperi-
    toneum, 132
  pretied loop, 4
  for retraction, 107, 108f
  through-and-through, for bleeding con-
    trol, 128f, 129, 130
Suturing, 137
  alternatives, 141–142
  hand-eye coordination, 139–140
  instruments, 140
  port positioning, 137–139, 138f
  training programs, 142–143
  visual perception and, 139–140
SVR (systemic vascular resistance), 189,
    202
Sword fighting, 87, 91f, 92
Syphilis, laparoscopic identification, 2
Systemic vascular resistance (SVR), 189,
    202

T

Tactile sensation feedback
  aids, 246
  in laparoscopic surgery, 80
  limited, 199
Target area, 16
Team, surgical, 155
Teleoperation, 244, 245f, 246–247
Television monitors. *See* Monitor(s)
Tension pneumothorax, 202
T-fasteners
  features, important, 44–45, 45f
  use, proper, 104, 106f, 106–107
Thermal noise, 18
Thermocoagulation, 4
Thiopental, 194
Thoracic procedures, operating room set-
    up, 159, 160f
Thoracoscopy, 17
  history of, 8
  imaging equipment, *73–74*
  indications, *73*
  one-lung ventilation for, 196
  operating space, maintaining, 74
  performing, 74–75
  special requirements, *73–75*
  therapeutic, 8
Through-and-through suture, for bleeding
    control, 128f, 129, 130
Tip-to-tip tissue approximation method,
    111, 112f
Tissue
  dissection, 120–121, 122f
  electricity effects on, 57, 58f–59f
  handling, 120–121, 122f
  laser effects on, 64–65
  removal techniques, 125–126
  retrieval devices, 126, 127f
Tissue approximation, 126–127
  partial staple deployment method, 111,
    113f
  tip-to-tip method, 111, 112f
  X arrangement, 111, 112f

Tissue morcellators, 55
Tissue retrieval devices, 54–55, 55f
Touch confirmation, 100, 140
Traction, 85, 86, 88f–89f
Training, 225–232
  animals for, 228–229
    methods/limitations, 230
    specific procedures in pig, 229–230
  didactic instruction, 226
  in humans, 231–232
  laparoscopic cholecystectomy, 7
  simulation for, 247–248
  in suturing, 142–143
  technology role, 230–231
  virtual reality, 230–231
  in vitro, 227–228
Transesophageal echocardiography, 189,
  194
Transperitoneal surgical approach, 237
Trendelenburg position, 3, 86
  for hernia repair, 174
  steep, 202, 205
  steep reverse, 162–163, 163f
  trocar insertion and, 95, 96f
  ventilatory parameters and, 190
Triangulation of ports, 137–138, 138f
Trocar(s), 3, 89. See also Trocar-cannula
    apparatus
  abdominal wall bleeding, 208
  bladder injuries, 207
  blind insertion method, 32
  with blunt obturator, 3
  bowel injuries, 207
  insertion
    closed technique, 94–98, 96f
    zigzag technique, 208–209
  liver injuries, 207
  mesentery injuries, 207
  placement, 132
  reusable, 32
  safety shields, 95, 205
  self-retaining collar, 97
  site
    bleeding, 208
    herniation, 208–209

risk of tumor/microorganism seeding,
  125
  tumor recurrence, 216
  spleen injuries, 207
  for thoracic surgery, 74
  vascular injuries, 206–207
Trocar-cannula apparatus, 29–32, 30f–31f,
  157
  anchor feature, 29–30
  safety feature, 29, 30f
Troubleshooting. See under specific problems
Trumpet valve, spring-loaded, 31f, 32
Tubal sterilization, by endocoagulation, 4
Tuberculosis, 2
Tumor biopsy, 4
Tumor recurrence, at trocar sites, 216
Tumor reduction therapy, 4
Twist knot, 150
Two-handed surgery (single-surgeon
    technique), 87, 89
Two-surgeons technique, 87

U

Ultrasound, 55–56, 75
  blood vessel detection, 121
  diagnostic, 67–69, 68f
    applications, 68–69
    probes, 67–68, 68f
    problems, 69
  dissector
    handpiece, 70–71, 72f
    specification, 70–71
  guidance, biopsy, 5
  probes
    frequencies used, 68
    high-frequency, 68
    linear scanning, 67, 68f
    low-frequency, 68
    mucosa-air interface, 69
    sector scanning, 67
  therapeutic, 61f, 69–71, 72f
    amplitude of vibration, 70, 71f
    cavitation and, 70

cutting devices, 71
  instrument specification, 70–71, 72f
Upper abdominal procedures, operating
    room set-up, 159, 160f
Upper airway obstruction, 197
Ureter injuries, 215
Urinary catheterization, 194
Uterine perforations, staging and repair
    of, 4

V

Vagal nerve injuries, 217
Vagina, cul de sac, 125
Vagotomy, 235
Vaporization, tissue, 57
Vascular injuries, from Veress needles or
    trocars, 206
Vascular procedures, thoracoscopic, 238
VCR (video recorder), 165, 178
Vecuronium, 195
Vena cava puncture, 206
Venous tamponade, 128
Veress needle, 3, 157
  abdominal wall bleeding, 208
  bladder injuries, 207
  blind obturator, 27–28, 28f
  bowel injuries, 207
  bowel penetration, 203
  insertion, 92–93, 203
  length, 170, 170t
  liver injuries, 207
  malposition, 169–170
  mesentery injuries, 207
  placement, confirmation of, 93
  spleen injuries, 207
  vascular injuries, 206–207
  visceral injuries, 205
Video camera, 157
Video endoscopic surgery, development
    of, 5
Video-guided laparoscopic surgery, 6
Video imaging equipment, 5, 139, 157
  design features, 13, 14f–15f, 16–17

set-up, 177, 177f
stereoscopic, 21
thoracoscopic surgery, 73–74
two-dimensional, technical complica-
    tions, 199, 200t
Video printers, 24
Video recorder (VCR), 165, 178
Videos, educational, 227–228
Video signal, 20
  compatibility with monitor/recording
      equipment, 21
  improper termination, 180
  monitor line input and, 177
  termination, 23
Virtual environments (virtual reality),
    230–231, 247–248
Viscera, needle in, pneumoperitoneum
    establishment and, 170, 170t
Visual field, brightness of, 19
Visual perception, hand-eye coordination
    and, 139–140

W

Water, as chromophore, 64
Western knot (Aberdeen knot), 151, 152f
White balance, 19
Windscreen washer-type device for lens
    system, 17
Wound infections, postoperative, 209,
    215

X

Xenon lamp, 23
X tissue approximation method, 111,
    112f

Y

Y-adapter, 27
Yankauer sucker, 74
Y/C signal, 20, 23